SEPARATION ANXIETY
IN CHILDREN AND ADOLESCENTS

Separation Anxiety in Children and Adolescents

AN INDIVIDUALIZED APPROACH
TO ASSESSMENT AND TREATMENT

ANDREW R. EISEN
CHARLES E. SCHAEFER

Foreword by David H. Barlow

THE GUILFORD PRESS
New York   London

For Linda, Zachary, and Carly–continuous sources of inspiration
For Great Aunt Mumi
and in beloved memory of my Great Uncle Manny
For the charter members of my fan club

—A. R. E.

For my family–Anne, Karine, and Eric–
for their unwavering love and support

—C. E. S.

© 2005 The Guilford Press
A Division of Guilford Publications, Inc.
72 Spring Street, New York, NY 10012
www.guilford.com

Printed in the United States of America

This book is printed on acid-free paper.

Last digit is print number: 9 8 7 6 5 4 3 2 1

Library of Congress Cataloging-in-Publication Data
Eisen, Andrew R.
  Separation anxiety in children and adolescents: an individualized approach to assessment and treatment / by Andrew R. Eisen, Charles E. Schaefer.
    p. cm.
  Includes bibliographical references and index.
  ISBN 1-59385-131-6 (hardcover: alk. paper)
  1. Separation anxiety in children. 2. Separation anxiety in adolescence. 3. Parent and child. I. Schaefer, Charles E. II. Title.
  RJ506.S46E37 2005
  618.92′ 8522–dc22
                                                    2004026091

About the Authors

Andrew R. Eisen, PhD, is Associate Professor in the School of Psychology/Sociology and Director of the Child Anxiety Disorders Clinic at Fairleigh Dickinson University. His research and clinical interests include childhood anxiety and related problems, nonverbal learning disorders, and sensory integration issues. Dr. Eisen is coauthor of *Practitioner's Guide to Treating Fear and Anxiety in Children and Adolescents: A Cognitive-Behavioral Approach* (1995, Jason Aronson) and coeditor of *Clinical Handbook of Anxiety Disorders in Children and Adolescents* (1995, Jason Aronson). He also has private practices focusing on children and families in Bergen County, New Jersey, and in Rockland County, New York.

Charles E. Schaefer, PhD, is Professor of Clinical Psychology at Fairleigh Dickinson University. He is also Director Emeritus of the International Association of Play Therapy and has coauthored or coedited more than 50 books on child therapy, play therapy, and effective parenting, including *Short-Term Play Therapy for Children* (2000, Guilford Press). In addition, Dr. Schaefer maintains a private practice in child psychology in Hackensack, New Jersey.

Foreword

It was not until the 1960s that psychotherapy began to deviate from a common and relatively uniform approach to treating psychopathology by tailoring treatments to specific psychological problems. Until that time the nature of psychopathology was ill defined and played little role in treatment planning. This changed rather dramatically during the 1970s and 1980s, beginning with the treatment of anxiety disorders and spreading across the full range of psychopathology as these problems became better delineated. It was, perhaps, DSM-III that first defined these concepts in enough detail to spark more broad-based attempts at designing treatments, both psychological and pharmacological, that would be especially effective in addressing the psychopathology at hand (Barlow, 1988). Ironically, the trend in the specification of treatments was more observable for what some are now calling "psychological treatments" (Barlow, in press) than for pharmacological treatments as individual treatment protocols appeared during the 1980s and 1990s for each of the disorders first articulated in DSM-III.

This trend began with Wolpe's (1958) description of systematic desensitization and continued in the 1970s with detailed descriptions of exposure-based treatments (Agras, Leitenberg, & Barlow, 1968; Marks, 1971). Systematic desensitization in particular sparked a flurry of research aimed at dismantling the effective ingredients in this well-operationalized procedure, and assessing with ever more precise measures the outcomes of this treatment. This in turn allowed psychotherapy investigators to begin refocusing research from an emphasis largely on process to one on outcomes (Barlow & Hersen, 1984; Hersen & Barlow, 1976). These developments resulted in a very healthy process in which theories of mechanisms of action in psychotherapy could be directly tested and modified or discarded in favor of more parsimonious and productive theories (Barlow, 1988). In this way, our science and practice began to complement one another in an iterative process resulting in newer and more effective treatments.

At the same time, great strides were occurring in our understanding of the nature of psychological disorders that, in turn, led to refinements in our treatment procedures. For example, one controversy in the early 1970s, referred to in the pages that follow in this book, explored the functional relationship of anxious behavior upon separation from parents in young children. One early study clearly delineated that the behavior of anxious separation could be a function of very different circumstances. For example, some young children might envision substantial harm coming to their parents or themselves during separation, which could be the focus of intense anxiety. Other children, upon careful analysis, were not actually anxious about separating per se, but found the school situation in all its complexity to be particularly anxiety provoking (Lazarus, Davison, & Polefka, 1965). This is not surprising in retrospect, but it was considered a very clever analysis at the time, which led directly to differential treatment planning.

It was this type of discovery in the clinical arena, as well as more basic phenomenological or phenotypical observations on presenting symptoms, onset, course, and response to treatment, that led to ever greater delineation and demarcation in our nosology, a tendency known as "splitting." Indeed, most investigators would agree that the field reached the zenith of splitting with the publication of the fourth edition of the *Diagnostic and Statistical Manual of Mental Disorders* (American Psychiatric Association, 1994) and its emphasis on reliably identified but very narrow slices of psychopathology resulting in numerous disorders (Brown & Barlow, 2002). More recently, experimental psychopathologists, nosologists, and therapy outcome researchers have begun to converge on a new conception of psychopathology that emphasizes commonalities rather than differences. This is particularly true in the emotional disorders, of which separation anxiety disorder is one. These new arguments point to findings reflecting substantial comorbidity among the emotional disorders as well as phenotypic similarity. Additionally, investigators have observed wide-ranging effects of treatments that were designed for specific disorders, such as phobia or depression, on accompanying comorbid emotional disorders where the therapeutic results are often as good as for the principal disorder. This indicates a possible nonspecificity of treatment, both psychological and pharmacological. Also underscoring commonalities among these disorders is emerging research on the latent structure of dimensional features of emotional disorders.

More recently, reflecting many of these developments from basic neuroscience to treatment outcome, we have proposed a theory of the etiology of emotional disorders referred to as "triple vulnerabilities" (Barlow, 1991, 2000, 2002), explicated in some detail in this book. The triple vulnerability theory encompasses a generalized biological vulnerability sometimes referred to as "temperament." This biological vulnerability involves nonspecific genetic contributions to the development of anxiety and negative affect. In the anxiety disorders, research has focused on such concepts as "anxiety," "neuroticism," "negative affect," or, particularly in the case of children, "behavioral inhibition." While each of these concepts has generated somewhat independent bodies of research, it is very likely that each concept is tapping, at least partially, a common theme associated with a biological vulnerability to developing emotional disorders generally.

A second vulnerability, referred to as a "generalized psychological vulnerability," comprises early-life experiences, often but not always traumatic or disruptive, that produce a sense of uncontrollability over important environmental events. This sense of uncontrollability seems to be at the core of negative affect and the derivative states of anxiety and depression (Barlow, 2002). Once again, a robust line of research from a variety of species, including humans, supports the salience of certain early-life experiences in shaping our views of the world or providing a filter for our experience. These two vulnerabilities alone, if they occur together, are likely to produce a generally anxious or depressive temperament if triggered by life events that may first manifest as separation anxiety and, later, as generalized anxiety disorder or depressive disorders. A third vulnerability, referred to as a "specific psychological vulnerability," is also a function of early experience, such as modeling from parents, and serves to focus anxiety on specific objects or situations, such as learning that certain animals or insects, certain somatic sensations, or social evaluations, are dangerous. The development and interaction of these diatheses has been outlined in some detail elsewhere (Barlow, 2002; Bouton, Mineka, & Barlow, 2001). What is important for the purposes of this book is that we are becoming more sophisticated in our understanding of the nature of psychopathology, allowing the development of more powerful and important treatments as described in this outstanding new effort from Andrew R. Eisen and Charles E. Schaefer.

The age of evidence-based treatments is upon us. Recently, governments and health care policymakers around the world have decided that many psychological treatments have evidence that is more than sufficient for inclusion in health care systems. This is very important because organized health care systems, faced with inadequate health care and spiraling costs, have decided that the quality of health care should improve, that it should be evidence-based, and that it is in the public interest to ensure that this happens (Barlow, in press; Institute of Medicine, 2001). Of course, our treatments, while demonstrably effective based on all the current rules of evidence, are far from perfect. Many individuals suffering from emotional disorders at clinically significant levels either fail to benefit from our treatments or improve only partially. Thus, we need a great deal more evidence on patient–treatment matching and on generalizing or translating robust results from psychological laboratories and clinics to the front lines where most clinical care is delivered.

It is also crucial that we develop more concerted efforts focused on early intervention and prevention. In this regard, as Eisen and Schaefer point out, separation anxiety has been considered in the past to be a risk factor for the later development of emotional disorders in adolescence and adulthood. This view is now not as popular as it once was, since it is very likely that separation anxiety is simply an early manifestation of the diatheses described previously, and that separation anxiety does not occur only in childhood, but can occur in adolescence and even in adulthood. Nevertheless, our best evidence is that early intervention with anxious or depressed children is not only effective but may introduce resilience to the development of later emotional disorders. For these reasons, the program developed by Eisen and Schaefer is particularly noteworthy in that important preventive purposes might be served in addition to the relief of current suffering.

In this age of evidence-based care, Eisen and Schaefer have developed a state-of-the-art, evidence-based treatment program for separation anxiety that draws not only on the latest thinking from the laboratories of cognitive and behavioral science but also on recent trends in research that emphasize prescriptive approaches and patient–treatment matching. These clinicians and scientists, experts in both fields, draw on years of experience to produce a treatment program that should bring us to the next level of clinical care for this very distressed population of children and their parents.

DAVID H. BARLOW, PhD
Director, Center for Anxiety and Related Disorders
Boston University

REFERENCES

Agras, W. S., Leitenberg, H., & Barlow, D. H. (1968). Social reinforcement in the modification of agoraphobia. *Archives of General Psychiatry, 19,* 423–427.

American Psychiatric Association. (1994). *Diagnostic and statistical manual of mental disorders* (4th ed.). Washington, DC: Author.

Barlow, D. H. (1988). *Anxiety and its disorders: The nature and treatment of anxiety and panic.* New York: Guilford Press.

Barlow, D. H. (1991). Disorders of emotion. *Psychological Inquiry, 2,* 58–71.

Barlow, D. H. (2000). Unraveling the mysteries of anxiety and its disorders from the perspective of emotion theory. *American Psychologist, 55,* 1247–1263.

Barlow, D.H. (2002). *Anxiety and its disorders: The nature and treatment of anxiety and panic* (2nd ed.). New York: Guilford Press.

Barlow, D. H. (in press). Psychological treatments. *American Psychologist.*

Barlow, D. H., & Hersen, M. (1984). *Single case experimental designs: Strategies for studying behavior change* (2nd ed.). New York: Pergamon Press.

Bouton, M. E., Mineka, S., & Barlow, D. H. (2001). A modern learning-theory perspective on the etiology of panic disorder. *Psychological Review, 108,* 4–32.

Brown, T. A., & Barlow, D. H. (2002). Classification of anxiety and mood disorders. In D. H. Barlow, *Anxiety and its disorders: The nature and treatment of anxiety and panic* (2nd ed., pp. 292–327). New York: Guilford Press.

Hersen, M., & Barlow, D.H (1976). *Single case experimental designs: Strategies for studying behavior change.* New York: Pergamon Press.

Institute of Medicine. (2001). *Crossing the quality chasm: A new health system for the 21st century.* Washington, DC: National Academy Press.

Lazarus, A. A., Davison, G. C., & Polefka, D. (1965). Classical and operant factors in the treatment of a school phobia. *Journal of Abnormal Psychology, 70,* 225–229.

Marks, I. M. (1971). Phobic disorders four years after treatment: A prospective follow-up. *British Journal of Psychiatry, 129,* 362–371.

Wolpe, J. (1958). *Psychotherapy by reciprocal inhibition.* Stanford, CA: Stanford University Press.

Preface

Fear of trying causes paralysis. Trying causes only trembling and sweating.
—MASON COOLEY

We are living in the "age of anxiety" (Spielberger & Rickman, 1990). Indeed, anxiety disorders are the most common mental health problems affecting children and adolescents. Separation anxiety is the most common of these disorders (5–10%), with as many as 41% of youngsters reporting issues of separation anxiety (Costello & Angold, 1995). Yet a paucity of specific treatment programs is available to help these youngsters and their families.

THE NEED FOR A COMPREHENSIVE SEPARATION ANXIETY TREATMENT PROGRAM FOR CHILDREN AND ADOLESCENTS

The development of this treatment program stemmed from three key factors. First, we called upon our more than three decades of combined clinical work with separation-anxious youth and their families. Second, despite the recent advances in treating anxious youth, treatment outcome efforts with separation-anxious youngsters seriously lagged behind. We believe this lag could be attributed to the perception of separation anxiety as any of the following:

- Product of early childhood.
- Normative developmental phenomenon that most youngsters outgrow.

- Variant of school refusal behavior.
- Result of faulty parent–child interaction patterns.

For these reasons, we began our own research efforts to better understand the nature and treatment of separation anxiety in children and adolescents.

Third, too few child clinicians are well versed in cognitive-behavioral therapy and how to treat the complexities of separation anxiety and related problems. As a result, we decided to develop a specific program for children and adolescents, with the following goals in mind:

- Distinguish separation anxiety from school refusal behavior.
- Identify separation anxiety as a challenging and often debilitating problem that may occur across the lifespan.
- Encompass multidimensional influences (i.e., biological, psychological, and psychosocial) involved in the development and maintenance of separation anxiety.
- Provide clinicians with step-by-step guidelines on how to treat the variety of separation anxiety presentations.

We drew from our clinical work and research as the well as the clinical research efforts of renowned experts, including David H. Barlow, Aaron T. Beck, Thomas H. Ollendick, Philip C. Kendall, and Wendy K. Silverman, to develop our own approach and treatment program. This book represents the culmination of these efforts.

WHO SHOULD USE THIS BOOK?

This book is suitable for doctoral- and master's-level therapists (with or without background in cognitive-behavioral therapy), school psychologists, social workers, licensed professional counselors, and graduate students with varied theoretical backgrounds. Our clinical material is extremely comprehensive and detailed, so that both novice and seasoned therapists can determine the level of guidance that is necessary for any given case. Our aims were three-pronged:

- Provide sufficient theoretical framework and developmental underpinnings for therapists with limited background in cognitive-behavioral therapy.
- Provide comprehensive knowledge of assessment measures and cognitive-behavioral therapy procedures, so that therapists can

implement them for a range of anxiety and related problems in children and adolescents.

- Provide step-by-step guidelines for working with children and adolescents (ages 3–17) experiencing a variety of separation anxiety issues.

ORGANIZATION OF THE BOOK

Part I: Introduction

In Chapter 1 we discuss the nature of separation anxiety and related problems and introduce our conceptual framework, which emphasizes specific symptom dimensions and safety signals. In Chapter 2 we discuss the normative experience of separation-related fears, the roles of attachment and temperament in the development and maintenance of separation anxiety, and the link between separation anxiety and panic.

Part II: A Prescriptive Approach to Assessment and Treatment

In Chapter 3 we introduce our prescriptive approach to assessing and treating children and adolescents with separation anxiety. A prescriptive approach uses empirically supported assessment measures to identify and match specific client characteristics with the most compatible and effective interventions. We show you how to implement this approach using standard measures in the field as well as with our newly developed Separation Anxiety Assessment Scale. We take you through the child and parent intake process in a step-by-step fashion, providing comments and clinical tips to help you proceed smoothly along the way. Here we also introduce the first of five case examples to address each of the dimensions of our prescriptive model.

Part III: Teaching Child Coping Skills

Chapters 4 and 5 provide step-by-step guidelines for teaching and practicing child coping skills (relaxation and cognitive therapy/problem solving). We show you how to prescriptively select different cognitive-behavioral exercises based on a youngster's dimension(s) of separation anxiety. Clinical tips, comments, and ample therapist–child dialogue will help you master the delivery of these skills across the varied separation anxiety presentations, comorbid conditions, and developmental levels.

Part IV: Teaching Parent Coping Skills

Chapters 6 and 7 provide step-by-step guidelines for teaching and practicing parent coping skills (education and contingency management). We show you how to prescriptively select different parent training exercises based on levels of parenting stress, competence, and anxiety. Clinical tips, comments, and ample therapist–parent dialogue will help you understand and work effectively with the variety of parenting styles you may encounter.

Part V: Confronting Separation Anxiety

Chapters 8 through 10 provide a step-by-step guide to treating the varied presentations of separation anxiety in children and adolescents across school, camp, and other settings. We provide an intricate narrative of the process of behavioral exposure to help you anticipate and prepare for therapeutic nuances as treatment unfolds. Maintaining a youngster's perception of control, modifying safety signals, and overcoming resistance are emphasized.

Part VI: Navigating the Obstacle Course

In Chapter 11 we show you how to help children and their families stay in control despite pitfalls and relapse. We discuss the challenge of comorbidity and problematic treatment implementation issues. We also consider the merits of pharmacotherapy, address termination issues, and introduce relapse prevention exercises.

Appendices

Appendices I and II provide assessment instruments and treatment-related handouts that will help you successfully implement our prescriptive approach.

GETTING THE MOST OUT OF THE BOOK

As a first step, we recommend that you carefully read the entire book before beginning treatment with any given case. It is important that you become fully familiar with the following factors:

- The variety of separation anxiety presentations in children and adolescents.

- The differing parenting styles and the challenges they pose.
- How to assess the dimensions of separation anxiety.
- How to treat the dimensions of separation anxiety.
- How to handle special obstacles (e.g., developmental constraints, comorbidity, treatment implementation issues).

Prior to conducting intake with a child who is separation anxious and his or her parent, review Part I to be prepared to answer any general questions regarding the nature and development of separation anxiety. Focus on Chapter 3 and decide which prescriptive assessment measures you will utilize. At the very least, we recommend that you employ our Separation Anxiety Assessment Scales (SAAS; see Appendix I). If you are familiar with, or have an interest in, some of the standard measures discussed, check the references for information on how to obtain these scales.

Following the intake, use your clinical judgment, the SAAS, and any of the assessment measures to determine the dimensions of separation anxiety, maintaining conditions, treatment recipients, and treatment approaches to be utilized. At that point, carefully review Parts III and IV and outline your treatment plan.

The next step is to select the case example in Part V that best exemplifies your current case and follow our step-by-step guidelines. As obstacles emerge, review Chapter 11 for helpful suggestions. Repeat this process for each new relevant case.

WHAT TO EXPECT

We assume that most children and their families will show moderate-to-marked improvement with this treatment. Many of our clients do experience complete remission of their separation anxiety symptoms. These families are typically quite motivated by, and dedicated to, the treatment process and face few special challenges. Even when youngsters are resistant, complete remission can occur, as long as you have the full support of the parents. Separation anxiety has one of the highest recovery rates with cognitive-behavioral therapy. Despite such positive treatment outcomes, a youngster's sensitivity to anxiety remains and may reappear in the future in a similar or different form (e.g., panic, generalized anxiety, depression). Thus our emphasis is on managing rather than curing separation anxiety and related problems. We recommend periodic follow-up visits and booster sessions.

Many of the families with whom you work will present with special challenges. To help you navigate the myriad issues and obstacles you are likely to encounter, we have provided five comprehensive case examples. We also provide a detailed narrative to guide you every step of the way. You may find that many of our case examples are more challenging than you typically encounter. If so, simply review the material that is most relevant. In this age of managed care, families may not seek treatment for their youngsters until their separation anxiety causes significant interference. About 10% of the children are likely to experience some residual separation anxiety. In complex scenarios you may have to help families adjust their ideas of realistic treatment outcomes. Few families fail to benefit; nevertheless, premature dropouts do occur occasionally, usually due to a parent's inability to follow through.

As you read this book, it may surprise you to learn just how much effort is required by a family to facilitate positive treatment outcomes. We will show you how to keep families motivated and vested in the treatment process. Mason Cooley's quote, "Trying causes only trembling and sweating, " is our motto. Your goal is to help youngsters and their families take small steps and work through the sweat. Together, one family at a time, clinicians and the families we work with can short-circuit the cycle of separation anxiety and subsequent problems.

Acknowledgments

We thank our students—Helen Raleigh, Lisa Brien, Charles Neuhoff, Lisa Hahn, Jennifer Hajinlian, and Jackie Mesnik—for their enthusiasm and dedication to the Separation Anxiety Treatment Project. Special thanks to Donna Pincus for her collaboration and shared vision. We are indebted to Kathryn Moore, Executive Editor of The Guilford Press, for her indispensable support, guidance, and encouragement throughout every phase of this work.

I (A. R. E.) want to thank my wife, Linda, for graciously taking care of our family the numerous times I needed to write, for her unceasing love and support, and for reading every word of this book and giving me encouraging feedback. You are the shining force that makes everything possible. This book is as much yours as it is mine. Special thanks to Cal and Phyllis Engler for being the charter members of my fan club. Words could not express what you mean to me. With love, admiration, and respect, I co-dedicate this book to you.

I (C. E. S.) want to thank my parents and my clients.

ANDREW R. EISEN
CHARLES E. SCHAEFER

Contents

INTRODUCTION

Part I lays the foundation for an individualized approach to assessment and treatment. In Chapter 1 we discuss the nature of separation anxiety and its related problems. More importantly, we introduce our conceptual framework, which emphasizes specific symptom dimensions rather than heterogeneous disorders. In Chapter 2 we discuss the normative experience of early separation-related fears and anxieties as well as developmental processes (i.e., attachment and temperament) that have relevance for clinical separation anxiety and panic responses.

CHAPTER I

The Nature of Separation Anxiety

> I remember playing outside alone as a child. Now, I can't get myself to
> leave my son with a babysitter. My husband wants to get a surveillance
> system. My friends are thinking about it too.
>
> —CONCERNED PARENT

THE PHENOMENON OF SEPARATION ANXIETY

Nothing seems safe these days. It's not surprising, given the ubiquitous
threats to our personal safety from terrorism, war, school killings, and
natural disasters. Imagine contracting *E. coli* from swimming in a public pool or Lyme disease from playing outside decades ago in "your"
day. Such environmental dangers are of great concern today (Rosen,
1998; Sloan, 1996), and for good reason. Understandably so, youngsters are experiencing more anxiety than ever before (Twenge, 2000).

Youngsters worry, and not just about environmental dangers.
School performance, social problems, or health-related issues can easily become daily preoccupations. In large-scale community surveys, as
many as 41% of children and adolescents reported separation concerns
(Costello & Angold, 1995). The most frequent and highest rated concerns reported involved personal safety and injury (56%; Silverman, La
Greca, & Wassertein, 1995), being alone (26%; Farach, 2002), and
sleeping alone (51%; Farach, 2002).

Separation-related worries (i.e., calamitous events to self or others;
getting sick) have also been shown to be prevalent in children who
engage in both internalizing (29%) and externalizing (20%) samples
(Barrios & Hartmann, 1997; Perrin & Last, 1997; Weems, Silverman, &
La Greca, 2000). In our own work (Hajinlian et al., 2003), we have

found that separation fears are common not only in children who have DSM-IV (American Psychiatric Association, 1994) anxiety disorders but attention-deficit/hyperactivity disorder (ADHD) as well. In fact, youngsters with ADHD reported greater percentages of fear around being alone and sleeping alone than youngsters experiencing a wide range of anxiety disorders (see Table 1.1).

Throughout the book we suggest that case formulations should emphasize these key fear dimensions. First, however, let's take a look at the nature of separation anxiety disorder (SAD), given that the bulk of the extant literature is based on this condition.

DESCRIPTION AND PREVALENCE OF SEPARATION ANXIETY DISORDER

Description

The central feature of SAD is unrealistic and excessive anxiety upon separation or anticipation of separation from major attachment figures (American Psychiatric Association, 1994, 2000). Primary symptoms include excessive worry about potential harm to oneself (e.g., getting kidnapped) and/or major attachment figures (e.g., car accident), nightmares involving themes of separation, and somatic complaints (e.g., stomachaches, headaches, vomiting).

Youngsters may avoid situations that lead to separation from primary caregivers and/or safe places. Common situations include refusing to attend school, be alone, sleep alone, or be dropped off at a friend's house or social event (e.g., party). Youngsters may resort to oppositional behaviors (e.g., temper tantrums, screaming, pleading,

TABLE 1.1. Prevalence of Separation Fears across DSM-IV Disorders

Separation fear	SAD (n = 18)	Other Anxiety (n = 17)	ADHD (n = 21)
Being alone	75%	31%	50%
Sleeping alone	83%	50%	56%
Being abandoned	83%	63%	50%

Note. SAD = separation anxiety disorder; Other Anxiety = generalized anxiety disorder, social anxiety disorder, obsessive–compulsive disorder, panic disorder, adjustment disorder with anxiety; ADHD = attention-deficit/hyperactivity disorder.

threats) when avoidance of the dreaded scenario becomes unlikely. As a result, parental accommodations (i.e., allowing youngsters to avoid) are common and ultimately can strengthen the separation anxiety response.

Epidemiology

Prevalence estimates for SAD in community samples range from 3 to 13% for children (Anderson, Williams, McGee, & Silva, 1987; Bird et al., 1988; Cohen, Cohen, & Brook, 1993) and from 1.8 to 2.4% for adolescents (Bowen, Offord, & Boyle, 1990; Cohen et al., 1993; Fergussen, Horwood, & Lynsky, 1993; McGee, Feehan, Williams, & Anderson, 1992). SAD onset is most common during childhood (ages 7–12 years; Compton, Nelson & March, 2000; Last, Perrin, Hersen, & Kazdin, 1992), with marked declines of onset during mid-adolescence and young adulthood. Nevertheless, SAD continues to affect individuals throughout the lifespan. For example, in a sample of college students SAD was associated with adjustment problems, eating disorders, and the onset and maintenance of depressive disorders (Ollendick, Lease, & Cooper, 1993). In child and adolescent anxiety disorder clinics SAD has been found to be as high as 47% (Last, Hersen, Kazdin, Finkelstein, & Strauss, 1987).

In general, SAD tends to be observed more frequently in girls than boys (Compton et al., 2000; Last, Hersen, et al., 1987; Last et al., 1992). However, boys may be more likely to be brought to mental heath professionals. The nature of separation anxiety symptoms (e.g., fear of being alone) may be viewed as more socially undesirable in boys, thus prompting families to seek help more readily (Compton et al., 2000).

RATES AND PATTERNS OF COMORBIDITY

Anxious youth frequently present for treatment with comorbid disorders (Verduin & Kendall, 2003). In fact, 79% were found to have at least one other disorder (Kendall, Brady, & Verduin, 2001). In this section we review the co-occurrence of SAD with other anxiety disorders, depression, school refusal behavior, and behavioral and learning disorders.

Generalized Anxiety Disorder

Generalized anxiety disorder (GAD) co-occurs in youngsters who have SAD approximately one-third of the time (Kendall et al., 2001; Masi, Mucci, Favilla, Romano, & Poli, 1999). This finding is not surprising, given that both disorders are associated with frequent worry and somatic complaints. By definition, however, the focus of worry in GAD is not limited to calamitous events to self or others, and its course is more chronic in nature (Cantwell & Baker, 1989; Masi et al., 1999). Separation anxiety may develop subsequent to GAD, if a youngster's experiences (e.g., a car accident involving a parent) or perceptions (e.g., neighborhood robbery) threaten his or her personal safety. When the disorders co-occur, SAD should be the initial focus of treatment if the threat of being alone or abandoned accounts for the greatest interference in functioning.

Obsessive–Compulsive Disorder

Recent research also reports the co-occurrence of obsessive–compulsive disorder (OCD) and SAD in children and adolescents. Although prevalence estimates for these two disorders typically range between 4 and 7% (Brynska & Wolanczyk, 1998; Spence, 1997), rates for SAD have been found to be as high as 24–34% in patients with OCD (Geller, Biederman, Griffin, Jones, & Lefkowitz, 1996; Valleni-Basile et al., 1994). The combination of OCD and SAD is also associated with an earlier onset of panic disorder (Goodwin, Lipsitz, Chapman, Manuzza, & Fyer, 2001).

Clinically, youngsters with both SAD and OCD may avoid being alone due to preoccupation with images of harm to themselves or others. OCD is associated with compulsions to neutralize the anxiety, whereas SAD is associated with excessive need of safety signals (e.g., safe persons, objects). When the disorders co-occur, features of both can be targeted concurrently. If the OCD is too severe, however, negotiating SAD as a first step may help build the momentum for managing the OCD symptoms.

Panic Attacks

Although panic disorder (PD) typically emerges during young adulthood (Burke, Burke, Regier, & Rae, 1990), panic attacks may be observed in children and adolescents with SAD. For example, in one study antecedent or associated separation anxiety was reported in 73% of youngsters (ages 7–18 years) who had panic attacks (Masi, Favilla, Mucci, & Millepiedi, 2000). In addition, a number of case reports has suggested that children, in general, may experience cued panic symptoms (e.g., Garland & Smith, 1991; Vitiello, Behar, Wolfson, & McLeer, 1990). However, these occasional, discrete experiences should be differentiated from PD, which involves recurrent panic attacks, uncued by the environment, as well as worries about having additional attacks (American Psychiatric Association, 1994). Concern regarding the implications of panic attacks (e.g., fear of dying, losing control) is generally not characteristic of children younger than 12 years of age (Kearney & Silverman, 1992; Nelles & Barlow, 1988). Hence, panic attacks in youngsters tend to be associated with physical (e.g., stomachaches, hyperventilation) rather than cognitive manifestations of anxiety. Separation-induced panic attacks tend to be associated with fears of abandonment and/or getting sick (Hahn, Hajinlian, Eisen, Winder, & Pincus, 2003).

Using structured interviews and questionnaires, prevalence estimates for PD in adolescence range from less than 1% (e.g., Wittchen, Reed, & Kessler, 1998) to greater than 10% (Hayward, Killen, Kraemer, & Taylor, 2000; Hayward, Killen, & Taylor, 1989), respectively. The most common symptoms reported include heart palpitations, trembling, dizziness, difficulty breathing, sweating, chest pain, and fear of dying.

Other Anxiety Disorders and Depression

Other anxiety disorders likely to coexist with SAD include social (8.3%) and specific phobias (12.5%; Kendall et al., 2001; Last, Hersen, et al., 1987; Verduin & Kendall, 2003). Youngsters who meet diagnostic criteria for posttraumatic stress disorder (PTSD) may also experience separation anxiety symptoms (e.g., refusing to be alone, school refusal behavior). However, such symptoms would be considered part of a PTSD diagnosis (Fischer, Himle, & Thyer, 1999). Given the association between anxiety and depression in children (e.g., Brady & Kendall, 1992), it's not surprising to find that SAD is frequently comorbid with depression. Approximately one-third of youngsters experience both SAD and a depressive disorder (Last, 1991; Last, Hersen, et al., 1987).

School Refusal Behavior

School refusal behavior is highly comorbid with SAD (Egger, Costello, & Angold, 2003). In fact, as many as 75% of children with SAD may also experience some form of school refusal behavior (Kearney, 2001; Last & Strauss, 1990; Masi, Mucci, & Millepiedi, 2001). In most cases, however, the school refusal behavior is acute, limited to mild forms (e.g., pleas to stay home, visits to nurse), and may not necessitate treatment.

Alternatively, chronic school refusal behavior is less likely to be associated with SAD. Rather, depression, panic, and agoraphobia, as well as other incapacitating conditions are often evident (Berg & Jackson, 1985; Kearney, 1993, 2001). Careful assessment can help distinguish the function(s) of school refusal behavior (see Kearney, 2001; Kearney & Albano, 2004).

Behavioral and Learning Disorders

Behavioral disorders are also likely to coexist with SAD. For example, ADHD (16.7%), oppositional defiant disorder (16.7%), and enuresis (8.3%) were found to be the most frequent comorbid disorders with SAD (Kendall et al., 2001; Last, Hersen, et al., 1987). Youngsters with a learning disorder (LD) are at risk for experiencing anxiety, depression, poor academic performance, and low self-esteem (e.g., Ialongo, Edelsohn, Werthhamer-Larrson, Crockett, & Kellam, 1994; Lyon, 1996). The presence of an LD may further diminish a youngster's perception of control. When an LD co-occurs with SAD, strong safety needs often emerge (see Chapter 11).

DIAGNOSTIC CONSIDERATIONS

As with any classification system, the categorical approach of DSM-IV is not without shortcomings. Both developmental and diagnostic limitations should be considered when using DSM-IV criteria to diagnose children and adolescents with SAD.

Regarding the developmental domain, no distinction is made between childhood and adolescent symptoms of separation anxiety. Rather, an early onset is noted if the diagnosis is assigned before age 6. This criterion is problematic because the nature, frequency, and intensity of separation anxiety symptoms often differ across the lifespan. For example, whereas the fear of being alone may appear at any point across the lifespan (e.g., Wijeratne & Manicavasagar, 2003), the fear of abandonment is strongest in younger children. Similarly, younger children are more likely to experience primarily somatic complaints, whereas older children and adolescents are more likely to experience both cognitive and somatic symptoms as well as a proneness to panic. Therefore, specific separation-related symptoms may offer differential prognostic value based on the frequency and intensity of the symptoms as well as their developmental origins.

Using DSM-IV criteria for SAD, a youngster must manifest any three (of eight) symptoms to qualify for a diagnosis. But it is not clear that all the symptoms are equivalent prognostic indicators. As a result of this artificial threshold (Frances, Widiger, & Fyer, 1990), some youngsters who are experiencing significant separation anxiety may fail to meet diagnostic criteria. It is important to keep in mind that family disruption can occur even when a youngster's separation anxiety is limited to one symptom (e.g., refusing to sleep alone at night).

In addition, the threshold problem (i.e., presence or absence of diagnosis) may obscure the heterogeneity that occurs within SAD. For example, some youngsters who experience separation anxiety are primarily concerned with being alone; others, with possible abandonment or getting sick (Eisen, Raleigh, & Neuhoff, 2003). A diagnosis of SAD, by itself, provides minimal information about the nature and intensity of the disorder. The one-month impairment criterion of DSM-IV is a step in the right diagnostic direction, because young children often experience developmentally appropriate separation anxiety that is transitory in nature (Rutter, 1981).

The overlap of disorders at both the symptom and diagnostic levels may also limit the usefulness of a SAD diagnosis. For example, at the level of the symptom, worry (Perrin & Last, 1997; Weems et al., 2000) and somatic complaints (Beidel, Christ, & Long, 1991; Last, 1991) are characteristic of emotional disorders in youth and are present to varying degrees in normative samples of youngsters (Egger, Angold, & Costello, 1998; Silverman et al., 1995). At the level of the disorder, SAD is frequently comorbid with both internalizing and externalizing disorders. Given these points of intersection, at times, it remains unclear as to which disorder is primary and should be addressed first (Eisen & Kearney, 1995).

KEY SYMPTOM DIMENSIONS

In general, given the limitations of DSM-IV and the frequent diagnostic comorbidity of disorders, there has been movement toward examining key symptom dimensions for specific adult (Barlow, 2002; Brown, Chorpita, & Barlow, 1998) and childhood internalizing problems (Chorpita, Albano, & Barlow, 1998; Eisen & Silverman, 1993, 1998; Kearney, 2001). In our work we have found that separation anxiety may be best understood by examining several key symptom dimensions that may account for separation-related symptoms individually or in combination and include fear of being alone (FBA), fear of abandonment (FAb), fear of physical illness (FPI), and worry about calamitous events (WCE; Hahn et al., 2003).

The first two dimensions directly capture the avoidance component of separation anxiety. The common fears associated with being alone and being abandoned are presented in Table 1.2.

TABLE 1.2. Fears of Being Alone and Abandoned

Being alone	Being abandoned
Living room	School
Family room	Carpool/bus
Bathroom	Play date
Bedroom	Extracurricular activity
Upstairs	Babysitter
Basement	Party
Attic	Parental errand
Kitchen	Sleep-over

Fear of Being Alone

Youngsters may be afraid to be left alone in certain areas of the house and therefore become the parent's shadow. Keep in mind that, in most cases, the FBA is strong even when a family member remains somewhere in the house. Daytime fears may include being alone in any room in the house or being on a different floor from other family members. At times, youngsters may be able to tolerate being alone if distracted by schoolwork, reading, television, or video games. Sometimes, however, distraction is not enough, especially if the entertainment system is in a more remote region of the house (e.g., finished attic or basement).

It is often easier for youngsters to be alone during the day than at night. Refusal to sleep alone is our most common referral. Youngsters who are afraid to sleep alone tend to have difficulty being alone during their nighttime routine as well. This may include going to the bathroom to brush their teeth or take a bath/shower, or simply settling down in their bedroom. As a result, bedtime may become a nightmare for the entire family.

If a youngster's separation anxiety is limited to FBA, his or her social and academic functioning outside of the home is typically unaffected. As long as the youngster is in the company of others, his or her perception of control generally remains intact. Compared to FBA, FAb tends to wield a broader influence and is more likely to threaten the nature of a youngster's academic and peer relationships.

Fear of Abandonment

Youngsters who fear abandonment may avoid certain places unless promised close proximity to a parent or major caregiver; for example, they may refuse to take the school bus or to be dropped off at a play date, extracurricular activity, birthday party, or sleep-over. During the preschool years, a parent may routinely stay with his or her youngster during these events. However, as elementary school progresses and greater independence from family members is expected, it becomes the norm for youngsters to separate from parents. Youngsters with FAb may fiercely protest any parental attempts to force separation, and/or they may make excuses to avoid attending the events on their own. Social isolation is often the result if avoidance becomes routine.

FAb may also have untoward effects at home. For example, youngsters may vehemently protest being left with a babysitter or resist a parent's efforts to run an errand. Unlike FBA, having family members present (e.g., older sibling) is not enough to quell a youngster's anxiety. Rather, the fear is specifically directed at the primary caregiver and the possibility of not being reunited with him or her.

Somatic Complaints/Fear of Physical Illness

The second set of dimensions—FPI and WCE—help to maintain a youngster's separation anxiety. The common somatic complaints/fears and worries associated with separation anxiety are presented in Table 1.3.

Epidemiological surveys have suggested that between 10 and 30% of children and adolescents report frequent headaches, stomachaches, and muscle/joint pain (e.g., Alfven, 1993; Egger et al., 1998). The ubiquity of somatic complaints has also been demonstrated in samples of

TABLE 1.3. Common Somatic Complaints/Fears and Worries

Somatic complaints/fears	Worries
Headaches	Harm to self or others
Stomachaches	Health of others
Dizziness	Being unable to cope
Fatigue	Getting lost/being abandoned
Feeling uncomfortable	Getting sick
Feeling sick	Being alone/sleeping alone
Choking	Disasters
Having an accident	Future events

Note. Somatic complaints based on Egger, Costello, Erkanli, and Angold (1999) and Last (1991); worries based on Farach (2002), Silverman, La Greca, and Wassertein (1995), and Weems, Silverman, and La Greca (2000).

children with childhood anxiety disorders, in general, and SAD, in particular (e.g., Beidel et al., 1991; Bernstein et al., 1997; Egger et al., 1999; Last, 1991).

For youngsters with separation anxiety, somatic complaints are usually in response to anticipated separations and will decrease when the threat of separation is removed. Sometimes the physical symptoms are exaggerated to gain attention or postpone separation (Eisen & Kearney, 1995). In general, however, it is not the experience of the somatic complaints, per se, but what they represent that maintains the youngster's separation anxiety. For example, a stomachache or nauseous feeling upon separation may trigger the fear of getting sick.

Although the youngster's fear may be limited to one or two somatic sensations (e.g., vomiting, choking) and there may not be evidence of cognitive symptoms (e.g., fear of dying, losing control; Nelles & Barlow, 1988), the youngsters may avoid situations or places that trigger these somatic cues. This dynamic, termed "interoceptive avoidance" (Barlow, 2002), is characteristic of panic disorder in adults.

As children get older and cognitive belief systems begin to develop, FPI may become associated with heightened anxiety sensitivity (AS; Reiss, Silverman, & Weems, 2001). Youngsters with elevated AS worry about the consequences (e.g., getting sick, losing control) of their bodily sensations. AS is associated with separation anxiety, school refusal behavior, and panic attacks (Kearney, 2001; Rabian, Peterson, Richters, & Jensen, 1993). FAb, however, tends to be maintained by a youngster's worry about calamitous events to others.

Worry about Calamitous Events

Common worries in youngsters include harm to self (e.g., being kidnapped, killed, or abandoned) or others (e.g., heart attack, serious accident, death; Perrin & Last, 1997; Silverman et al., 1995; Weems et al., 2000). WCE may maintain FBA, especially if youngsters are worried about bad things happening to them at home (e.g., getting sick, burglar intrusion). As youngsters venture out to the world, however, WCE (to others) typically maintains FAb.

For example, a fear of not getting picked up at school is often fueled by a fearful preoccupation with possible catastrophic injury to the primary caregiver. Any sign of lateness on the caregiver's part may easily spiral a youngster's anxious apprehension. As a result, youngsters will often avoid a variety of separation-related situations unless promised close proximity to the caregiver. When separation does occur, as is inevitable, these youngsters are convinced that disaster has been averted only after reunion.

SAFETY SIGNALS

Given the nature of separation anxiety symptoms, it's not surprising that youngsters cling to safe persons, places, transitional objects, or actions during anticipated separations. Safety signals help individuals feel more secure and may lead to the perception of restored personal control in anxiety-provoking situations (Barlow, 2002; Craske, 1999). Common safety signals associated with separation anxiety are presented in Table 1.4.

Safety signals are frequently present across the dimensions of separation anxiety and related disorders (Hajinlian et al., 2003) and can easily allay a youngster's anxious apprehension. For example, regarding FBA, being with others augments the youngster's perception of personal safety (e.g., help is available if physical sickness develops) and minimizes preoccupation with the potential occurrence of calamitous events to self or others. Transitional objects (e.g., "blankie") and favorite activities (e.g., watching television, playing video games) also enhance a youngster's feelings of security when caregivers are unavailable.

Overall, it is important to keep in mind that safety signals can serve useful functions (e.g., as a lucky charm, so to speak) and at times may be considered developmentally appropriate. At the same time, however, excessive reliance on safety signals may serve to strengthen a youngster's separation anxiety (i.e., through avoidance behavior) and thereby result in a limited range of functioning in social and academic

TABLE 1.4. Common Safety Signals for Youngsters with Separation Anxiety

Persons	Places	Objects	Actions
Primary caregiver	Home	Night light	Calling a parent
Parent/ guardian	Relative's house	"Blankie"	Eliciting specific promises
Relative	Best friend's house	Special toy	"Shadowing" the caregiver
Sibling/pet	Parent's room	Stuffed animal	Sleeping with others
Best friend	Sibling's room	Book	Staying with the nurse
Teacher/ nurse/coach	Familiar place	Food/drink	Engaging in favorite activity

areas. The gradual elimination of unhealthy safety signals coupled with the learning of new coping strategies are considered integral to facilitating successful treatment outcome in separation-anxious youth.

SUMMARY

Separation anxiety disorder is characterized by unrealistic and excessive anxiety upon separation or anticipation of separation from major attachment figures. Given the diagnostic limitations of DSM-IV and the frequent comorbidity of SAD with other disorders, it may be best to examine the key symptom dimensions of FBA, FAb, FPI, and WCE. Careful attention must also be paid to the number, frequency, and intensity of safety signals developed by an anxious youngster. Our dimensional framework sets the stage for identifying and implementing prescriptive treatment strategies.

CHAPTER 2

Development of Separation Anxiety

As a child I was afraid of everything: school, being alone, the dark, you
name it. I always felt sick to my stomach when I had to leave the house.
My mother said I was a sensitive child. My father tried to toughen me up.
It didn't work. Nothing did. No one knew what was wrong with me. I'm 42
years old now, and I have panic attacks. My 4-year-old is just like me.
                                                              —CONCERNED PARENT

NORMATIVE DEVELOPMENTAL PHENOMENA

As the above example illustrates, it is becoming painfully clear that
childhood separation anxiety can have devastating consequences for
years to come. In this section, we discuss the nature and course of early
forms of distress (i.e., separation, strangers, fears) that may have implications for the development of separation anxiety and panic.

Separation Distress and Stranger Anxiety

Separation distress and stranger anxiety are considered largely innate,
universal phenomena that occur in humans as well as many other species (Marks, 1987; McKinney, 1985; Mineka, 1982). Individual differences exist in the amount of distress displayed during infancy and
toddlerhood and are likely the result of biological vulnerabilities
(Plomin & Rowe, 1979). Separation distress and stranger anxiety are
considered distinct phenomena for several reasons. For example, separation distress, characterized primarily by infant crying in response to
parental separation, emerges as early as 4 months (Ainsworth, 1967;
Kagan, Kearsley, & Zelazo, 1978) and typically peaks around 13–18
months (Bowlby, 1973; Campbell, 1986). Stranger anxiety, characterized by crying, fear, and escape behaviors, emerges around 7 months

(Thompson & Limber, 1990) and peaks around 12 months (Plomin & Rowe, 1979). The most fundamental difference between the two is that separation distress is believed to be a form of protest (i.e., anger), whereas stranger anxiety more closely resembles the experience of fear or panic (Emde, Gaensbauer, & Harmon, 1976; Shiller, Izard, & Hembree, 1986). As a result, stranger anxiety may have more salient implications for the development of clinical separation anxiety (see Barlow, 2002).

It is important to keep in mind that most infants typically experience minor and transient forms of separation distress and stranger anxiety that usually fade within the second and third years of life (Menzies & Harris, 2001). This pattern should be distinguished from clinically significant separation anxiety that emerges around 4 or 5 years of age.

Separation-Related Fears

Separation-related fears begin during the first year of life and typically persist until 7 or 8 years of age (e.g., separation from caregivers, being alone, the dark). Most of these fears tend to be mild and transient and may have protective functions. Fears that have limited impact and last less than 1 month are likely part of normal development or the result of a precipitating event. However, fears that emerge during expected developmental intervals may still necessitate intervention if they are intense or persistent enough to significantly interfere with family life, school, or peer relationships.

The course for separation anxiety generally follows a developmental progression. For example, younger children tend to experience fewer and less distressing symptoms, whereas older children and adolescents experience greater avoidance levels and frequent somatic complaints and worries (Francis, Last, & Strauss, 1987; Last, 1991). Although most youngsters negotiate separation anxiety, for others, symptoms may continue into adolescence and adulthood (Manicavasagar, Silove, & Curtis, 1997; Manicavasagar, Silove, Curtis, & Wagner, 2000). If still evident during young adulthood, greater adjustment problems are likely, compared to individuals who reported experiencing separation anxiety only as children (Ollendick et al., 1993).

DEVELOPMENTAL PROCESSES

In this section we discuss developmental processes that have implications for how infants and children manage separations, strangers, and exploratory activities. Each process may protect against, or increase the risk of, separation anxiety and related problems. We emphasize the roles of attachment and temperament in the development and maintenance of separation anxiety.

Attachment

Attachment is an enduring emotional tie between the infant and his or her caregiver that sets the stage for individual adaptations (Bowlby, 1969, 1982). The security of the attachment relationship is believed to be associated with the quality of caregiving (Bowlby, 1969, 1982). Characteristics of caregivers that appear to promote secure mother–infant relationships include sensitivity, positive attitude, synchrony, mutuality, support, and stimulation (DeWolff & van IJzendoorn, 1997).

Youngsters with secure attachments are more likely to be self-confident and trusting in their close interpersonal relationships, display better social skills, and experience fewer negative emotions (Englund, Levy, Hyson, & Sroufe, 2000; Kochanska, 2001) than their insecurely attached counterparts. Secure relationships have protective value and may help to immunize youngsters from developing later separation anxiety and related problems (Spence, 2001). The majority (i.e., 65%; Shaffer, 2002, p. 397) of infants and toddlers are classified as having secure attachments with their mothers.

Alternatively, insecure mother–infant attachments are believed to result from insensitive and/or inconsistent caregiving (Isabella, 1993). A number of studies with anxious youth has characterized their families as higher in control and conflict and lower in warmth and support than the families of children who do not have internalizing problems (Baumrind, 1989; Dumas, LaFreniere, & Serketich, 1995; Siqueland, Kendall, & Steinberg, 1996; Stark, Humphrey, Crook, & Lewis, 1990). Such family environments may result in a diminished sense of personal control in the youngster (Sroufe, 1990) and may facilitate the development of a generalized psychological vulnerability (Fonagy et al., 1996) characterized by an insecure-ambivalent/resistant attachment.

Separation anxiety may be associated with insecure-ambivalent/resistant (anxious) parent–child attachments (e.g., Main, Kaplan, & Cassidy, 1985; Ollendick, 1998). Preliminary research has shown a relationship between insecure-ambivalent/resistant (anxious) attachment styles and child and adolescent anxiety disorders (Cassidy & Berlin, 1994; Cowan, Cohn, Pape-Cowan, & Pearson, 1996; Rosenstein & Horowitz, 1996; Warren, Huston, Egeland, & Sroufe, 1997). Furthermore, insecure-ambivalent/resistant attachments account for 15% of mother–infant dyads (Ainsworth, Blehar, Waters, & Wall, 1978).

Temperament

Temperament refers to an inherited tendency to react a certain way in both novel and challenging situations (Kagan, 1989, 1994). Thomas and Chess (1977) initially identified nine dimensions of temperament: activity level, rhythmicity (i.e., regularity of body functions), approach–withdrawal, adaptability, intensity, threshold (i.e., degree of responsiveness), mood, distractibility, and persistence of attention. These dimensions accounted for the three well-known patterns: easy, difficult, and slow-to-warm-up temperaments.

Easy temperament profiles (i.e., positive reactivity) are associated with greater adaptability and may have protective value in minimizing later risk for anxiety and related disorders. Approximately 60% of 1-year-olds are classified as having easy temperament profiles (e.g., Caspi, Henry, McGee, Moffitt, & Silva, 1995; Chess & Thomas, 1984).

Difficult temperament profiles (i.e., negative reactivity) are associated with school adjustment issues, aggressive behavior, and problematic family and peer relations (Lytton, 1990; Thomas, Chess, & Korn, 1982). In addition, difficult temperament profiles are associated with externalizing problems such as oppositional defiant disorder (ODD) and ADHD (Maziade et al., 1990). Slow-to-warm-up profiles are associated with a cautiousness to embrace novel or challenging situations (Chess & Thomas, 1984). Difficult and slow-to-warm-up profiles account for 15% and 23% of infants, respectively (Shaffer, 2002; Thomas & Chess, 1977).

The construct of behavioral inhibition (BI; Kagan, 1994, 1997) has the most relevance for the development of anxiety disorders, in general, and separation anxiety, in particular. In early childhood, BI often resembles separation anxiety and includes general fearfulness, cautiousness, irritability, and clinging/dependent behaviors. Infants and toddlers may withdraw from unfamiliar settings and persons and seek comfort from caregivers when distressed. Approximately 15–20% of 2-year-olds are classified as behaviorally inhibited (Kagan, 1989, 1994).

Evidence suggests that youngsters exhibiting BI are at increased risk of developing anxiety disorders (Anthony, Lonigan, Hooe, & Philips, 2002; Hirshfeld et al., 1992; Lonigan & Philips, 2001; Lonigan, Vasey, Philips, & Hazen, 2004). In addition, the degree of risk increases considerably if BI remains stable and one of the parents has an anxiety disorder (Biederman, Rosenbaum, Chaloff, & Kagan, 1995).

Goodness of Fit

The relationship between quality of caregiving and temperamental influence as each relates to attachment security remains a topic of fierce debate. Although the bulk of the literature supports maternal responsiveness as a key determinant of secure attachment relationships (e.g., DeWolff & van IJzendoorn, 1997; Isabella, 1994; Kochanska, 1998; Pederson & Moran, 1996), temperamental influence appears to have both direct (Seifer, Schiller, Sameroff, Resnick, & Riordan, 1996; van den Boom, 1994) and indirect (Calkins & Fox, 1992; Kagan, 1994) effects.

Thomas and Chess's (1977, 1986) goodness-of-fit model is a useful framework with which to consider the transactional relationship between the infant's response style (i.e., temperament) and his or her physical and social worlds (i.e., family environment). Both attachment security and temperament profile may change over time and are affected by contextual factors. For example, poor caregiver–infant temperament pairings could set the stage for separation anxiety. Caregivers may respond to their infant's inhibited temperament with overprotectiveness (Thompson & Calkins, 1996), overvigilance, or indifference and negativity (Kagan, Arcus, & Snidman, 1994). Each of these parental response styles may increase the risk of later separation anxiety and related problems (e.g., Bowen, Vitaro, Kerr, & Pelletier, 1995). In contrast, when caregivers provide their infants with a healthy balance of support, guidance, and autonomy, anxious reactivity may be minimized (e.g., Fox & Calkins, 2003).

In the following section, we examine the relationship between early separation anxiety and the development of panic disorder with agoraphobia (PD-Ag) in adulthood. We conclude the chapter with developmental models that highlight the roles of temperament and attachment in the etiology of both separation anxiety and panic.

DEVELOPMENTAL CONTINUITIES

A number of investigations (e.g., Ayuso, Alfonso, & Rivera, 1989; Breier, Charney, & Heninger, 1986; Klein, Zitrin, Woerner, & Ross, 1983; Laraia, Stuart, Frye, Lydiard, & Ballenger, 1994; Yeragani, Meiri, Balon, Patel, & Pohl, 1989; Zitrin, Klein, Woerner, & Ross, 1983; Zitrin & Ross, 1988) has supported the link between separation anxiety in childhood and panic disorder in adulthood. In general, these studies suggested that adult patients with PD-Ag had higher rates of separation anxiety as children, compared to other childhood disorders. However, these findings need to be interpreted with caution due to strong methodological constraints.

For example, the majority of studies was retrospective in nature, employed differing definitions of PD-Ag and SAD/school phobia, utilized unreliable assessment measures, and failed to account for diagnostic comorbidity. In addition, several studies either failed to demonstrate this association (e.g., Hayward et al., 2000; Thyer, Neese, Curtis, & Cameron, 1986) or suggested that SAD served as a risk factor for adult anxiety disorders, in general (Lipsitz et al., 1994; van derMolen, van der Hout, van Dieren, & Griez, 1989).

In an attempt to improve the retrospective assessment of SAD, Silove and colleagues (1993) developed the Separation Anxiety Symptom Inventory (SASI), a self-report measure designed to assess childhood experiences of separation anxiety. Using the SASI, Silove and colleagues (Manicavasgar et al., 2000; Silove & Manicavasagar, 1993; Silove et al., 1993, 1995) demonstrated that childhood separation anxiety was associated with a lifetime history of panic disorder. Recently, however, a 7-year longitudinal study (Aschenbrand, Kendall, Webb, Safford, & Flannery-Schroeder, 2003) reported that youngsters with SAD experienced no greater likelihood of developing PD-Ag in young adulthood than youngsters who had a range of other anxiety disorders.

Overall, it remains unclear whether SAD is exclusively associated with PD-Ag or represents a general risk factor for anxiety disorders in adulthood (Lipsitz et al., 1994; van derMolen et al., 1989). If specific separation anxiety dimensions (rather than heterogeneous cases of SAD) were examined over time, perhaps a more precise relationship between separation anxiety and PD-Ag would emerge. For example, based on our work with separation anxious youth, we would predict that FAb, maintained by FPI and a range of safety signals, would have the strongest association with PD-Ag. In forthcoming chapters (Chapters 8–10), we discuss how youngsters who have this profile share remarkable similarities with adults with PD-Ag.

DEVELOPMENTAL MODELS

Pathways to Separation Anxiety

Current developmental models suggest that both temperament and attachment play important roles in the etiology of anxiety disorders, in general, and separation anxiety, in particular. Rubin and Mills (1991) outlined a pathway to anxiety disorders stemming from the interaction of temperament, family socialization experiences, and contextual conditions (e.g., stress, poverty). Their model suggests that temperamental wariness indirectly influences the security of attachment. For example, an infant's high-intensity and fearful temperament may prompt the caregiver to become overprotective and overinvolved in attempts to soothe. As a result, the infant's bids for exploration become restricted and an insecure attachment may develop (Bowlby, 1973).

Lonigan and colleagues (Lonigan & Philips, 2001; Lonigan et al., 2004) proposed a model that highlights the importance of temperamental risk in the development of anxiety disorders. Drawing from work in personality theory, they suggested that high negative affectivity/neuroticism (NA/N) and low effortful control (EC) predisposes children directly or indirectly to anxiety. High NA/N is largely characterized by fear, discomfort, anger/frustration, and emotionality. The construct of EC is related to the ability to self-regulate mood and attentional processes (e.g., shifting, focusing, inhibitory control). Youngsters with anxiety disorders (i.e., low EC) may have difficulty shifting their attention away from distressing stimuli (for reviews, see Vasey & MacLeod, 2001).

Lonigan and Philips (2001) noted that these personality dimensions closely resemble a behaviorally inhibited temperament. According to their model, temperamental risk (high NA/N and low EC) may directly or indirectly (when combined with other processes such as attachment, conditioning, attentional biases) lead to the development of anxiety disorders. Separation anxiety may be more likely if youngsters fail to habituate to normal separation-related fears and/or stressful events.

Pathways to Panic

Ollendick and colleagues (Mattis & Ollendick, 1997; Ollendick, 1998) adapted Barlow's model (Barlow, 1988, 2002) to explain the development of childhood separation anxiety and its link with adult panic disorder. The model integrates biological and psychological vulnerabilities. For example, biological vulnerability may stem from a behaviorally inhibited temperament, characterized by heightened sympathetic nervous system activity under stress. Within this framework, the experience of separation may activate a strong neurobiological stress response (e.g., Rosenbaum, Biederman, Hirshfeld, Bolduc, & Chaloff, 1991).

Psychological vulnerabilities may stem from parent–child interaction patterns that lead to internal working models of the world (e.g., Bowlby, 1982) as unpredictable and uncontrollable. Ollendick suggests that an insecure-ambivalent attachment reflects the unpredictable and uncontrollable dimensions of the youngster's family environment and may help to explain the child's difficulties with the process of separating, exploring, and reuniting with the caregiver.

As biological and psychological vulnerabilities interact, heightened reactions to separation-anxious events may emerge. Further psychological vulnerabilities in the form of interoceptive conditioning and anxiety sensitivity (i.e., a focus on internal somatic cues), may maintain and intensify the cycle of anxious apprehension, ultimately leading to the development of panic and possible agoraphobic avoidance.

SUMMARY

The development of separation anxiety and its link to panic is firmly rooted in biological (temperament, anxiety sensitivity), psychological (attachment), and environmental (separation-anxious events) vulnerabilities. Helping youngsters negotiate the dimensions of separation anxiety begins with the process of a comprehensive assessment, described in Part II.

PART II

A PRESCRIPTIVE APPROACH TO ASSESSMENT AND TREATMENT

On the following pages, we present our prescriptive approach to assessing and treating youngsters with separation anxiety (Eisen et al., 2003; Eisen & Silverman, 1998; Neuhoff, Hahn, & Eisen, 2003). A prescriptive approach attempts to identify and match specific client characteristics with the most compatible interventions. Such an approach is becoming recognized as an effective way to facilitate positive treatment outcomes (Beutler, 1991; Chorpita, Taylor, Francis, Moffitt, & Austin, 2004; Hayes, Barlow, & Nelson-Gray, 1999; Kearney & Silverman, 1990, 1999).

In Chapter 3, for example, using empirically supported measures, we prescribe child and adolescent cognitive-behavioral interventions on the basis of cognitive and/or somatic symptoms. Thus, youngsters who are experiencing primarily separation-related worries would be given cognitive-based procedures. On the other hand, youngsters experiencing primarily somatic complaints (e.g., stomachaches, headaches) would receive relaxation-based procedures. Of course, youngsters experiencing both cognitive and somatic symptoms would receive a combination of treatment approaches. Using our newly developed Separation Anxiety Assessment Scale (SAAS; Hahn et al., 2003) we also demonstrate how to tailor your child- and/or family-based treatment according to the specific dimensions of separation anxiety.

Each of the cases in this book is based on a composite of youngsters with separation anxiety whom we have treated. Five case illustrations are presented to address each of the separation-anxiety dimensions of our prescriptive model. Our first case example, introduced in Chapter 3, involves a 7-year-old Caucasian boy, Brian, and his parents, Mr. and Mrs. P.

Assessing Separation Anxiety

My daughter has become so clingy. She won't let me go anywhere by myself. If I try, she holds her stomach and screams. She won't even visit her best friend in the neighborhood. She just sits in her room and cries. I don't know what's wrong. She was never like this before.

—CONCERNED PARENT

THE ASSESSMENT PROCESS

Separation anxiety is a heterogeneous emotional problem. Differences among youngsters can be observed regarding symptom dimensions, impact, maintaining factors, comorbid problems, and developmental levels. Therefore, a comprehensive assessment of separation anxiety and related problems should include information from a range of sources. In addition, keep in mind that the assessment process is both dynamic and ongoing. For this reason, it's important to monitor progress related to both process-related changes and treatment outcome with empirically supported measures.

In this chapter, we take you through the parent consultation and child intake process in a step-by-step fashion. Presenting complaints are discussed in relation to separation anxiety dimensions and DSM-IV diagnosis. Careful attention is devoted to *assessment tools* (empirical measures to supplement your inquiries), *data checks* (how to prescribe treatment that is consistent with empirical data), *data gathering* (early developmental experiences, family history, adverse events), *comments* (what to expect), and *clinical tips* (what should be discussed in session). In Dialogue 3.1, we begin with Mr. and Mrs. P.'s presenting concerns regarding their son, Brian, as reported during the parent consultation.

Brian, age 7, is terrified of being alone during the day and at night. He lives with his parents and two older sisters in a three-story house. During the day, Brian always needs someone to be with him. He avoids spending time in the family room or finished basement unless a family member is present. Brian constantly follows his mother or sister(s) around the house. He needs a family member to be on the same floor and close by so he can either see or hear them. He refuses to be in the bathroom alone to use the toilet or to brush his teeth. Most problematic, however, is his refusal to sleep alone at night. Brian responds with screaming, crying, and throwing himself on the floor when his parents insist that he sleep alone in his room.

PARENT CONSULTATION

Dialogue 3.1

MRS. P.: Brian refuses to sleep in his room at night. We're exhausted (*sighing and looking at her husband*). We don't know what to do anymore.

THERAPIST: What happens when you insist that Brian sleep in his room?

MRS. P.: He refuses. He gets very angry and throws himself on the floor. He keeps everyone up for hours.

MR. P.: It doesn't bother me when he sleeps downstairs.

MRS. P.: But it's not just at night. He follows me around all day. He can't even go to the bathroom by himself. Why is Brian like this?

THERAPIST: Every child comes into the world with a certain amount of sensitivity to anxiety.

MRS. P.: I knew it was our fault (*looking at Mr. P.*). He's always been such a sensitive child.

THERAPIST: It's no one's fault. And it's not a bad thing to be sensitive. Brian's sensitivity is what makes him loving, sweet, and affectionate. We would never want to change that. But because he *is* sensitive, sometimes he may worry too much or take everything personally. So the idea is to *retain* all of his wonderful qualities, and *contain* his anxiety.

MRS. P.: (*Lets out a deep sigh.*). Did we wait too long to get help for Brian?

THERAPIST: Not at all. Brian can learn to minimize his anxiety by applying the coping skills we will teach him. Each time you let

Brian visit you at night, you're taking away his anxiety and not giving him a chance to deal with it.

MRS. P.: But we want him to feel safe.

THERAPIST: Our goal is to help Brian learn to feel safe on his own.

Comment

Now the stage is set for a supportive and collaborative therapeutic alliance. You can continue gathering relevant information as the therapy proceeds. To ensure that your coverage is appropriately comprehensive, we recommend utilizing some form of structured interview.

STRUCTURED INTERVIEWS

Several structured interviews have been developed in both child and parent versions to assess child psychopathology, in general, and anxiety disorders, in particular. These include:

Diagnostic Interview Schedule for Children (DISC; Costello, Edelbrock, Dulcan, Kalas, & Klaric, 1984)

Schedule for Affective Disorders and Schizophrenia for School-Age Children (K-SADS; Puig-Antich, Orvaschel, Tabrizi, & Chambers, 1980)

Diagnostic Interview Schedule for Children and Adolescents (DICA; Herjanic & Reich, 1982)

Interview Schedule for Children (ISC; Last, Strauss, & Francis, 1987)

Child and Adolescent Psychiatric Assessment (CAPA; Angold & Costello, 2000)

Child Assessment Schedule (CAS; Hodges, Kline, Stern, Cytryn, & McKnew, 1982)

Children's Interview for Psychiatric Symptoms (Weller, Weller, Fristad, Rooney, & Schecter, 2000)

Anxiety Disorders Interview Schedule for DSM-IV (ADIS-C; Silverman & Eisen, 1992; Silverman & Nelles, 1988).

Anxiety Disorders Interview Schedule for DSM-IV

In general, each of these interview schedules possesses adequate psychometric properties (see Silverman, 1991). However, in our work with anxious youth, we employ the most recent version of the ADIS-C, which is based on the DSM-IV (Silverman & Albano, 1996). The ADIS-C and the ADIS-P (parent version) provide the most comprehensive coverage of DSM-IV anxiety disorders. In addition, the section on SAD covers anxiety symptoms and etiology, provides a functional analysis of the disorder, and even addresses early developmental precursors. The ADIS-C and ADIS-P also permit differential diagnosis of the majority of other child behavior disorders and/or problems.

Comment

The use of a structured interview certainly has its advantages. For example, excellent reliability has been demonstrated for the ADIS-P (Rapee, Barrett, Dadds, & Evans, 1994; Silverman & Eisen, 1992; Silverman, Saavedra, & Pina, 2001) and other interview schedules (e.g., Shaffer, Fisher, Lucas, Dulcan, & Schwab-Sone, 2000) for anxiety and related disorders. Based on the ADIS-P, parents were found to be excellent reporters of a youngster's SAD (Silverman et al., 2001). However, if you were to administer the ADIS-P (and ADIS-C) in its entirety, the intake would be extremely cumbersome. This is why structured interviews tend to be implemented in clinical research settings only. For your purposes, it might be better to draw from certain sections depending on the referral question. It would be helpful to be fully familiar with the content of the questions for SAD and related disorders. This way, your assessment would be diagnostically driven, in part.

Data Check

In Brian's case, the use of the ADIS-P facilitated a DSM-IV diagnosis of SAD. In addition to separation anxiety, Brian's parents expressed concern about his recent hand washing at night. Queries from the OCD section of the ADIS-P revealed that Brian did not meet criteria for this disorder. His rituals were not time consuming, nor did they interfere with his social and academic functioning. Rather, they appeared to be a consequence of his separation anxiety and helped "protect" him at night when alone.

GATHERING DEVELOPMENTAL DATA

Reconstructing a youngster's early developmental milestones is no easy task. Relatively accurate histories (i.e., pregnancy, birth, speech/language development, motor delays) are more likely to be obtained when complications have occurred. In general, your coverage should address demographics, pregnancy and birth, early developmental milestones (i.e., motor development, speech/language development, toilet training, eating, sleeping), school and medical histories, medications, and peer relationships. Developmental data can be collected as part of the parent consultation or in the form of a preevaluation (March & Mulle, 1998). To save time, consider sending the Conners–March Developmental Questionnaire (Conners & March, 1996) or Developmental History Forms (Freedheim & Shapiro, 1999) to the family soon after the consultation is scheduled.

The developmental information that is most relevant to a youngster's separation anxiety is listed in Table 3.1. Difficult early separation-related experiences, a family history of anxiety and related problems, and adverse events associated with separations from caregivers may increase a youngster's vulnerability to separation anxiety. What's important here is to relate a youngster's developmental history to the family's presenting concerns.

Data Check

Based on Brian's parents' report, his developmental milestones were within normal limits, and his birth, delivery, and medical histories were unremarkable. Mrs. P. reported that Brian had always been strong-willed, intense, and needy. Specifically, she described her son as overly fearful and cautious, easily frustrated, a picky eater, and a poor sleeper. She also reported that Brian had difficulty separating during preschool and experienced a difficult transition to first grade.

TABLE 3.1. Developmental Information Relevant to Separation Anxiety

Early experiences	Family history	Adverse events
Strangers	Emotional disorders	Hospitalizations
New situations	Separation anxiety/panic	Family losses
Preschool	Behavioral inhibition	Separation/divorce
Shyness/hesitancy	Insecure attachments	Remarriage
Sleeping alone	Treatment/medications	Relocations

Oppositional Features

In our experience, the majority of youngsters with separation anxiety have features of a behaviorally inhibited temperament. Brian was described as being fearful and cautious as well as having difficulty adjusting to novel situations. In addition, many youngsters also possess features of the "difficult" temperament profile. For example, Brian was described as strong-willed with low frustration tolerance. Keep in mind that you will likely address both separation anxiety and oppositional features during the treatment program.

PARENT-COMPLETED MEASURES

In addition to gathering developmental information, you may find it helpful to supplement your inquiries with salient parent-completed measures. In the next section, we provide an overview of some helpful measures to consider as part of your multimethod–multisource assessment. We address the following: separation anxiety, child behavior problems, temperament, attachment, parental psychopathology, and family environment.

Separation Anxiety

The Separation Anxiety Assessment Scale—Parent Version (SAAS-P) assesses the key dimensions of separation anxiety (as discussed in Chapter 1) and is presented in Appendix I with clinical norms and instructions for scoring. The four dimensions include Fear of Being Alone (FBA), Fear of Abandonment (FAb), Fear of Physical Illness (FPI), and Worry about Calamitous Events (WCE). In addition, the SAAS-P contains a Frequency of Calamitous Events (FCE) subscale as well as a Safety Signals Index (SSI). The FCE subscale is useful to determine if any actual precipitating events may have triggered the youngster's separation anxiety. Preliminary data support the psychometric utility of the scale (Hahn et al., 2003).

The Weekly Record of Anxiety at Separation (WRAS; Choate & Pincus, 2001) helps parents keep track of the frequency and intensity of their youngster's separation-related behaviors on a daily basis in the following areas: school, bedtime, play and other activities, parents' departure, parents' location, parents' well-being, and child's well-being. Some parents may view the WRAS as a bit cumbersome, because it covers such a broad range of separation-related situations. For this reason, consider administering only those sections deemed relevant for a particular youngster (see Handout 6 in Appendix II).

Data Check

Based on the SAAS-P, Brian's FBA largely accounted for his separation anxiety, and his FPI appeared to maintain his avoidance behavior. The FCE picked up precipitating triggers that included the death of Brian's grandfather and "hearing about bad things happening to people." Brian received low scores for FAb and WCE, suggesting only minor abandonment concerns or worries about calamitous events. The SSI revealed a number of safety signals, including family members, nightlight, "blankie," and familiar babysitters.

Child Behavior Problems

The Child Behavior Checklist (CBCL; Achenbach, 1991a) is a 118-item parent-completed measure that covers the range of internalizing and externalizing behavior problems. The CBCL also contains separate age and gender profiles, strong psychometric properties, and relies on a national normative base. Relevant subscales for assessing separation anxiety include Withdrawn, Somatic Complaints, and Anxious/Depressed.

The Conners Rating Scale—Parent Version Revised (CRS-PVR; Conners, 1997) is an excellent measure to consider, especially if there are time constraints (e.g., the short form contains only 27 items) or ADHD is likely a comorbid disorder. The CRS-PVR contains Oppositional and Hyperactive–Impulsive subscales as well as an ADHD index. Relevant subscales for assessing separation anxiety include Psychosomatic, Anxious-Shy, and Perfectionism.

Temperament

The Emotionality, Activity, and Sociability Temperament Survey (EAS; Buss & Plomin, 1984) is 20-item parent-completed self-report measure that assesses a youngster's temperament across five dimensions: distress, fear, anger, activity, and sociability. Recently, a modified youth version was developed (EAS-K; see Anthony et al., 2002). Sample items from the EAS-K include "I am easily frightened" and "I get emotionally upset easily."

The Child Temperament and Behavior Q-Set (CTBQ-Set; Buckley, Klein, Durbin, Hayden, & Moerk, 2002) is an observational measure that includes the characteristic temperamental dimensions but also contains a separation anxiety/dependency subscale. The CTBQ-Set is useful in home and school settings, but it is time consuming to administer. Specific separation-related items may be of value in your office setting.

Attachment

The Attachment Q-Set (AQS; Waters, Vaughn, Posada, & Kondo-Ikemura, 1995) consists of 90 descriptors of attachment-related behaviors. A parent, caregiver, or trained observer is asked to sort the descriptors in the youngster's natural environment. Attachment classifications based on the AQS have yielded results similar to the Strange Situation measure (Ainsworth et al., 1978).

Parental Psychopathology

We know that anxiety disorders can have a familial/genetic basis. A growing body of research suggests that offspring of parents with anxiety disorders are at risk for developing anxiety disorders themselves (e.g., Beidel & Turner, 1997; Biederman et al., 2001; McClure, Brennan, Hammen, & LeBrocque, 2001). In one study, 63% of children with SAD had at least one parent who experienced a general adult version of the disorder (Manicavasagar, Silove, Rapee, Waters, & Momartin, 2001).

Measures of parental psychopathology can help determine the impact of parental problems on child anxiety and related disorders as well as a parent's ability to participate in a family-based treatment program. To assess parental anxiety, consider administering the Beck Anxiety Inventory (Beck, 1993) or the Fear Questionnaire (Marks & Mathews, 1979). The Beck Depression Inventory–II (Beck, Steer, & Brown, 1996) and the Millon Multiaxial Clinical Inventory (Millon, Millon, & Davis, 1994) are helpful for assessing parental depression and personality disorders, respectively.

Family Environment

Additional measures of family dynamics can contribute to a multimethod–multisource assessment. The Family Environment Scale (FES; Moos & Moos, 1986) and the Family Adaptability and Cohesion Evaluation Scales–III (FACES-III; Olsen, 1985) both possess strong psychometric properties and can be used to assess the family environments of anxious youth. The FES contains 90 items and 10 subscales. Relevant subscales for assessing separation anxiety include Independence, Cohesion, Expressiveness, and Control. The FACES-III addresses the degree to which families are enmeshed, disengaged, separated, or neglected; research has suggested that separation anxiety is associated with enmeshed families (Kearney & Silverman, 1995; Pilkington & Piersel, 1991).

Data Check

Through a combination of relevant queries and parent-completed measures, additional information was obtained. Brian's frequent and intense somatic complaints as well as his oppositional behaviors (e.g., temper tantrums) were reported to be his most distressing behavior problems.

Mrs. P. reported that she also struggled with anxiety and panic attacks and was currently taking antianxiety medication. Mr. P. reported a family history remarkable for depression. Brian's family environment was characterized as high in control, based on both parents' report. Mrs. P., however, was best viewed as overprotective, controlling, and caring, whereas Mr. P. appeared somewhat disengaged. Finally, both parents discussed the impact of the passing of Brian's paternal grandfather 6 months prior to the consultation.

Clinical Tip

Many parents are concerned about the potential stigma of bringing their child to a therapist. Given that you will be implementing a cognitive-behavioral therapy program (Kendall, 2000), we find it most helpful to present yourself as a coach who will be teaching coping skills. Most parents find this approach comforting.

In addition, be sure to encourage parents to mention their session with you, as well as the idea of a coach, to their child *before* you conduct the child intake process. Overprotective parents who have separation-anxious youth may attempt to shield their children from distress. As a result, some youngsters may be unaware of the reason for their visit with you. Such conditions will likely exacerbate the issue of separation during the intake. Remember, parental overprotection may be prompted by a need to comfort the child; however, it may also be related to a reluctance or unwillingness to deal with a child's distress (see Chapter 6). In Dialogue 3.2., we discuss the coach concept with Mr. and Mrs. P.

Dialogue 3.2

MRS. P.: What should we say to him [Brian]? We're concerned he'll think he has problems. We don't want this to hurt his self-esteem.

THERAPIST: Tell Brian that I am a coach. I'll teach him skills, and then we'll apply them in different situations. We'll work together until Brian's confidence emerges, and both of you feel that you're becoming good at facilitating his coping.

MR. P.: I'm not sure if he'll buy into this.

THERAPIST: Does Brian play any sports?

MR. P.: Yes he does . . . basketball and baseball. He's a pretty good athlete. If only he didn't get so frustrated. He quits everything he starts (*with an exasperated sigh*).

THERAPIST: You can tell Brian that I'm an anger coach or a fear coach. Mention specific separation and anger-related situations with which he struggles. Ask him if he'd like some help in learning to calm down.

MRS. P.: I'd like to try [this program].

MR. P.: (*Nods*).

Homework

Toward the conclusion of the consultation, ask the parent(s) to prepare a brief list of problematic separation-related situations to give you at the time of the child intake sessions. The list should include situations that provoke anxiety, anger, and avoidance behavior. This list will be helpful when you meet the youngster as well as when you develop exposure hierarchies (see Chapter 8).

CHILD INTAKE

The child intake is typically more oriented toward developing rapport than the parent consultation, especially when assessing young children. When assessing older children and adolescents, use your judgment to achieve an optimal balance between data collection efforts and rapport-building activities.

An Informal Separation Anxiety Test

A youngster's reaction to parental separation during the intake is an important source of diagnostic and developmental data and provides hints of attachment classifications. Meeting with you for the first time, separating from a parent, and spending time alone with an unfamiliar professional are all potentially anxiety-provoking scenarios in the mind of a separation-anxious youngster.

In the Separation Anxiety Test (SAT; Greenberg, 1999; Hansburg, 1972; Klagsbrun & Bowlby, 1976; Shouldice & Stevenson-Hinde, 1992) a youngster typically responds to pictures depicting varying themes of separation from caregivers. The SAT is administered in the context of brief Strange Situation episodes. For our purposes, the intake represents an informal SAT and may be considered an authentic, in vivo (i.e., reality-based) exposure.

In our experience, most youngsters with separation anxiety will eventually separate from caregivers during the intake. Mild-to-moderate resistance is common. However, as you can imagine, some intakes are extremely difficult to negotiate and require a good deal of preparation.

Youngsters with insecure-ambivalent attachments are likely to pose the greatest challenge during the intake, exhibiting physical (e.g., clinging, grabbing, yelling, crying) and/or verbal (e.g., "Help," "Don't leave me") forms of separation anxiety. Keep in mind that such behaviors may be exacerbated if they also possess features of behavioral inhibition and/or "difficult" (e.g., strong-willed) temperamental characteristics. Remember, the combination of behavioral inhibition and an insecure-ambivalent attachment increases vulnerability to separation-anxious events.

Children ages 3–8 years who fear being alone may resist parental separation until they warm up to you. Typically, after two or three visits, they will separate comfortably. However, older children and adolescents may still forcefully resist parental separation if they fear abandonment. In this case, achieving a youngster's gradual separation from the parent in your office, the waiting area, and the building will be important targets for change during the treatment program.

Meeting Brian

In the waiting area, Brian was sitting next to his mother. Mr. P. was sitting adjacent to them, reading a magazine. The therapist introduced himself and then asked Brian if he'd like to talk for a little while. Immediately, Brian sat in his mother's lap, started to shake, and then held onto her forcefully.

DIALOGUE 3.3

MRS. P.: (*Trying to stay calm*) C'mon, Brian. We talked about this. He's a coach. He wants to help you be less scared when you're alone.

BRIAN: (*Crying, shaking*) I can't.

THERAPIST: Would you like to play a game?

BRIAN: No! I can't!

MRS. P.: Brian . . . please get off me. (*She tries to peel him off, but*

Brian only grabs her harder. She looks at her husband, who is still reading his magazine.)

MR. P.: (*Looking annoyed, he puts down his magazine.*) Brian . . . (*in a firm, loud voice*)

BRIAN: (*Looks up, stops shaking.*) My stomach hurts (*holding his stomach*).

MR. P.: (*Starts to get up.*)

THERAPIST: (*Gestures for Mr. P. to remain seated, starts to speak in a soft voice*) Brian, can you look at me?

BRIAN: (*Turns around, faces therapist.*)

THERAPIST: Brian, it's okay if you're scared to come in and talk with me. A lot of kids are. Would it help if Mom and Dad came in too?

BRIAN: (*Gives a half-smile, wipes his eyes, then nods in agreement.*)

Comment

The child intake should employ rapport-building activities such as playing games, talking about hobbies, and art projects. It is initially very important to help a separation-anxious child feel comfortable. The minimal goal should be to spend at least a few minutes alone with the youngster, even simply playing a game. There may be some negotiation, but you can gradually fade the parent(s) out of your office. If necessary, leave the door slightly ajar or have a parent sit outside, close to the door.

Create the expectation that during forthcoming visits, you will be meeting with the youngster alone. If you're unsuccessful on the first visit, don't despair. Be sure to tell the parents not to lose hope either. As the youngster warms up to you, it will be easier to implement firmer limits. Once the youngster willingly separates, following some rapport-building activities, you can begin to inquire about the nature of his or her separation anxiety and related problems.

Clinical Tip

During the child intake, present your own personally relevant example of a childhood fear or phobia. Using this example, you can help the youngster understand the relationship between fear and avoidance. By choosing your own personal example, you will serve as a coping model and help the youngster realize that everyone has fears. Be sure that your examples are concrete in nature (e.g., fear of dogs, planes, the dark). In Dialogue 3.4 we present a dog phobia example.

Dialogue 3.4

At this point, Brian is sitting in his own chair. Mr. and Mrs. P. are still present in the office.

THERAPIST: (*Looking at Brian*) I'd like to tell you a little story. When I was your age, I was afraid of dogs . . .

BRIAN: (*Interrupting and smiling*) I'm not afraid of dogs.

THERAPIST: That's great. Everyone is afraid of something (*Gestures to parents to contribute*).

MRS. P.: I don't like planes . . .

MR. P.: (*Smiles, remains silent.*)

THERAPIST: (*Looking at Brian again*) I lived on this nice cul-de-sac, and everyday I would go out and play with my friends. But one of my friends had a big black dog that roamed everyone's property. Whenever I saw her, I became really scared. So when no one was looking, I'd quietly walk away, then run into my house and slam the door. After a while, I stopped going outside.

BRIAN: How come?

THERAPIST: I thought the dog was going to bite me. Pretty soon, my friends stopped calling me. They didn't know I was afraid of the dog. They thought I didn't want to play with them anymore. Six months went by. I didn't have a *coach* to help me be less scared.

BRIAN: What did you do?

THERAPIST: (*Taking a deep breath*) Well . . . I decided that if I wanted to have friends, I'd have to go outside. So one day I stepped outside and waited by my doorstep. And sure enough, the black dog headed for my property. I stood there shaking, closed my eyes, and prayed that the dog wouldn't bite me. And you know what the dog did?

BRIAN: (*Anxiously anticipating answer, shrugs his shoulders.*)

THERAPIST: Sniffed me and walked away!

BRIAN: (*Smiles with relief.*)

THERAPIST: So you see, Brian . . . the only way to overcome anxiety is to experience anxiety. When the dog approached me, I *did get* very scared. But when I realized that nothing bad was going to happen, my fear went away. And you know what? From that day on, I was never again afraid of dogs.

BRIAN: (*Smiles.*)

Comment

The dog phobia example created a personal connection between Brian and his therapist. The next step was to help Brian relate the dog phobia story to his own experiences with separation anxiety. We illustrate this relationship in Dialogue 3.5.

Dialogue 3.5

THERAPIST: Brian, what do you think will happen when you're alone?

BRIAN: (*Shrugs his shoulders.*)

MRS. P.: You can tell him.

BRIAN: I don't know (*getting irritated*).

THERAPIST: Has anything bad happened when you were alone?

BRIAN: No . . . I don't want to talk about it.

THERAPIST: Is it your stomach?

BRIAN: (*Nods.*)

THERAPIST: What could happen?

BRIAN: I'll get sick.

THERAPIST: Have you been sick before?

BRIAN: No . . . but I could get sick.

THERAPIST: When I had nervous thoughts about the dog, did that mean the dog was going to bite me?

BRIAN: No.

THERAPIST: When your stomach feels upset, does that mean you will be sick?

BRIAN: I guess not.

THERAPIST: That's right. When your stomach feels funny, it's just your body's way of saying *you're scared.* So when you visit your mom and dad at night, you're doing the same thing that I did. You're running away from your fear. Just like when I ran into my house. So what do you need to show yourself?

BRIAN: That nothing bad will happen?

THERAPIST: That's right. And how will you do that?

BRIAN: By staying in my room.

THERAPIST: Great. We'll take small steps, and soon you'll be ready.

Comment

At this point, if a parent(s) is still present in your office, attempt to phase him or her out. Brian allowed his parents to sit in the waiting area as long as the office door was left ajar. His therapist agreed to play a game following a brief series of questions. Consider using some of the following assessment tools to augment your inquiries.

Structured Interview

When interviewing children and adolescents, we recommend drawing on relevant sections of the ADIS-C, depending on the referral question. The content of the questions for the SAD section is similar to the ADIS-P (e.g., "Do you feel really scared or worried when . . . ?") (Silverman & Albano, 1996) and is presented in a developmentally appropriate manner.

It is well documented that children and adolescents can reliably report their feelings using the ADIS-C (e.g., Rapee et al., 1994; Silverman & Eisen, 1992; Silverman et al., 2001) and other interview schedules (Ambrosini, 2000; Angold & Costello, 2000; Reich, 2000). Indeed, SAD tends to be one of the more reliable anxiety disorder diagnoses (Silverman et al., 2001).

Of concern, however, is the tendency for low correlations to emerge between adult and child reports of anxiety and related disorders (Rapee et al., 1994). For this reason, the use of multiple informants can increase the accuracy of your information. The consensus is that youngsters may still be the best reporters of their own emotional states (e.g., Aronen & Soininen, 2000). This view may be true even for children with SAD. However, depending on the child's age and the circumstances surrounding the referral, the time frame for collecting this information may extend well beyond the intake.

Data Check

Brian was initially cooperative about answering questions concerning school and friends. However, he kept looking toward the office door to ensure that his parents were still there. In addition, he repeatedly asked, "Is it time to play a game yet?" When the questions gradually shifted to inquiring about nature of his anxiety, Brian responded frequently with "I don't know." He began to hold his stomach and said that he needed to go to the bathroom. The therapist granted permission, then asked," Are you ready to play a game?" Brian suddenly perked up and moved toward the play area. During the game, the therapist asked brief questions about Brian's separation anxiety. Brian's responses were still limited, but he admitted to being afraid to be alone, especially at night.

Comment

When it comes to interviewing children and adolescents who have separation anxiety, it is important to be realistic about the kind of information you will gather during the intake. This is especially true when youngsters fear being alone or abandoned. For this reason, consider administering some of the following self-report measures to round out your intake.

CHILD SELF-REPORT MEASURES

Child self-report measures are useful tools that identify the specific nature of separation anxiety and related problems and help set the stage for prescriptive treatments. In the next section, we provide an overview of some useful measures (for youngsters ages 6–17 years) to consider as part of your multimethod–multisource assessment. The measures we describe address separation anxiety, physical and cognitive anxiety, generalized anxiety and fearfulness, as well as depression and behavioral problems.

Separation Anxiety

The Separation Anxiety Assessment Scale–Child Version (SAAS-C; developed by Eisen, Hahn, Hajinlian, Winder, & Pincus) is similar to the parent version regarding both the content and structure of the questions. The SAAS-C assesses the key dimensions of separation anxiety; it is included in Appendix I with clinical norms and instructions for scoring. FBA and FAb capture the avoidance component of separation anxiety. FPI and WCE are viewed as maintenance factors. The frequency of calamitous events (FCE) helps determine whether precipitating factors are contributing to a youngster's separation anxiety. Finally, the safety signals index (SSI) is useful for identifying treatment targets and the extent of avoidance behaviors.

The Multidimensional Anxiety Scale for Children (MASC; March, 1997) contains 45 items, possesses strong psychometric properties, and contains a separation anxiety subscale. Sample items include, "I get scared when my parents go away," "I try to stay near my mom and dad," "I sleep next to someone in my family," and "I keep the light on at night." The MASC is most useful for corroborating a diagnosis of SAD and helps identify youngsters who struggle with somatic complaints (e.g., the physical anxiety subscale).

The "What's Happening to Me?" daily diary (DD) helps youngsters to keep track of separation-related situations that provoke anxiety, anger, and avoidance behavior; see Handout 3 in Appendix II. Our emphasis during this point of the assessment process is to determine whether separation anxiety is manifested primarily as bodily symptoms, apprehensive cognitions, or both. Data from the DD will contribute to prescriptive treatment selection. Based on developmental considerations (e.g., youngster's age, willingness to self-monitor), use your judgment to determine the extent to which DD recording should become a family endeavor (e.g., each night a parent can help solicit and/or record relevant symptoms).

Physical and Cognitive Anxiety

The Revised Children's Manifest Anxiety Scale (RCMAS; Reynolds & Richman, 1978) contains 37 items, possesses strong psychometric properties, and yields four subscales: Worry/Oversensitivity, Physiological, Concentration, and Lie. Separation-related items include, "It is hard for me to get to sleep at night," "Often I feel sick to my stomach," "I wake up scared some of the time," "I worry when I go to bed at night," and "I often worry about something bad happening to me." Elevated scores on the Worry/Oversensitivity and Physiological indexes are most useful for assigning prescriptive treatments (e.g., relaxation training for somatic complaints, cognitive therapy exercises for worry; Eisen & Kearney, 1995; Eisen & Silverman, 1998).

The Child Anxiety Sensitivity Index (CASI; Silverman, Fleisig, Rabian, & Peterson, 1991) contains 18 items, possesses strong psychometric properties (e.g., Silverman et al., 1991), and measures how aversive children view the experience of physical sensations (e.g., "It scares me when I feel like I am going to throw up"). Many youngsters with separation anxiety are afraid to experience uncomfortable physical feelings such as stomachaches or headaches. Elevated scores on the CASI are characteristic of children who have a proneness to panic-like symptoms and later panic disorder (Kearney, Albano, Eisen, Allen, & Barlow, 1997). Relaxation-based procedures can help "shut off" the cycle of anxious apprehension triggered by uncomfortable physical feelings (Barlow, 2002; Eisen & Kearney, 1995; Eisen & Silverman, 1998).

Generalized Anxiety and Fearfulness

The State–Trait Anxiety Inventory for Children (STAIC; Spielberger, 1973) contains two 20-item scales that measure state (variable) and trait (stable or chronic) anxiety. Both scales possess strong psychometric properties (Spielberger, 1973) and contain relevant items for assessing separation anxiety (e.g., "I worry about my parents"). The trait version is particularly useful for disentangling comorbid generalized and separation anxieties. For example, elevated trait anxiety scores help corroborate a GAD diagnosis and suggest that separation anxiety may be temporary in nature and easier to negotiate during treatment (e.g., Eisen & Silverman, 1993, 1998; Eisen et al., 2003).

The Fear Survey Schedule for Children–Revised (FSSC-R; Ollendick, 1983) contains 80 items, possesses strong psychometric properties (Ollendick, 1983), and measures general fearfulness. Relevant items for assessing separation anxiety include positive (fear) responses to "Having to go to school," "Being alone," and "Being left at home with a sitter." The FSSC-R has been shown to discriminate youngsters with generalized anxiety from those who fear going to school (Last, Francis, & Strauss, 1989). Like the STAIC (trait), elevated scores are more characteristic of youngsters with GAD.

Depression and Behavioral Problems

Older children and adolescents who experience strong forms of separation anxiety and related problems are at risk for depressive symptoms. Among adolescents, major depressive episodes and dysthmia are often the result of strong avoidance behavior triggered by separation and generalized anxieties, panic attacks, and school refusal responses (Kearney, 2001; Kearney & Silverman, 1995).

Alternatively, young children's depression-like symptoms (e.g., crying, weepiness) may be more of a function of separation anxiety (e.g., attention getting, somatic complaints) and temperamental variation (e.g., low frustration tolerance) than a true mood disorder (Eisen & Kearney, 1995; Kearney, 2001). If depressive symptoms are evident, consider administering the Children's Depression Inventory (CDI;

Kovacs, 1992) or the Reynold's Child/Adolescent Depression Scale (Reynolds, 1989). Finally, with older children, if behavioral problems complicate the symptom picture, consider administering the Youth Self-Report (YSR; Achenbach, 1991b), which is appropriate for 11–18-year-olds, contains 118 items, strong psychometric properties, an extensive normative base, and assesses the full range of internalizing and externalizing behavior problems.

Data Check

Data from the child self-report measures provided support for a diagnosis of SAD and indicated the importance of physical anxiety as a maintaining factor. For example, based on the SAAS-C, Brian's separation anxiety was largely due to FBA and maintained by FPI. The FCE identified precipitating factors (i.e., grandfather's passing), and the SSI revealed a number of safety signals (e.g., his mother, siblings, nightlight, radio, "blankie"). Brian also scored in the clinical range on the separation anxiety subscale of the MASC. In addition, elevated scores for physical anxiety subscales were evident on a number of measures (i.e., MASC, RCMAS, CASI). Lastly, Brian did not report depressive symptoms.

Comment

When administering self-report measures, it is important to take into account the age of the youngster. For example, young children (i.e., ages 4–8 years) possess limited cognitive skills, are less likely to attend to emotional events, and may not fully appreciate the nature of their emotions (House, 2002). The measures we recommended are brief, concrete, and symptom oriented, and with guidance (i.e., reading or explaining questions) from a parent or professional, youngsters can contribute to the assessment process.

PRESCRIPTIVE TREATMENT PLANNING

The ADIS-C supported a DSM-IV diagnosis of SAD for Brian. The SAAS-C captured the nature of Brian's separation anxiety. For example, FBA (being alone) largely accounted for his separation anxiety fears and FPI (somatic complaints) maintained his avoidance. For these reasons, consistent with the child data, prescriptive relaxation-based procedures were recommended (Eisen & Kearney, 1995; Eisen & Silverman, 1998; Neuhoff et al., 2003) to help him manage the physical feelings in his body. Brian will also learn to use these strategies as coping tools in scenarios that provoke separation anxiety (see Chapter 4). The relaxation-based procedures will replace his need to stay close to family members (shadowing, oppositional behaviors) and/or cling to safety signals.

In addition, consistent with the parent data, prescriptive parent-training procedures were also recommended (Eisen, Engler, & Geyer, 1998; Eisen et al., 2003; Neuhoff et al., 2003). Through parent training (see Chapters 6 and 7), Mr. and Mrs. P. will learn to facilitate Brian's coping and become acutely aware of how their own actions (and inactions) inadvertently encourage his separation anxiety.

Clinical Tip

It is important to remember that during treatment, a youngster's separation anxiety is likely to *get worse before it gets better.* This is not surprising, given that most youngsters will only reluctantly give up parental comfort and safety signals. It takes time for youngsters to understand the need and value of prescriptive coping skills. Be sure to discuss this likelihood with parents *before* treatment begins, presenting it as part of the therapeutic process. Otherwise, some parents may perceive their youngster's resistance as evidence that the program is not working, become frustrated, and terminate prematurely.

PART III

TEACHING CHILD COPING SKILLS

In Part III we present guidelines for teaching and practicing child coping skills in a step-by-step fashion. Chapters 4 (relaxation) and 5 (cognitive therapy) are presented as independent modules, so that you can prescriptively select specific exercises based on a youngster's degree of separation anxiety, developmental level, and comorbid problems. In addition to presenting basic tools and procedures, we also include clinical tips, comments, and how-to sections.

Our second case example, introduced in Chapter 4, involves a 15-year-old Caucasian girl, Felicia, who fears being alone and abandoned. She lives with her parents in an older, Colonial-style house. Felicia's older brother is attending college in another state. Felicia has a strong fear of physical illness. For example, she is terrified of vomiting or becoming out of breath. Her respiratory concerns are partly related to a mild preasthmatic condition. Nevertheless, she is an avid but fearful participant on her high school track team.

Felicia's fear of being alone manifests largely at night. Given that both of her parents work during the day, she is adapting to staying home alone in the afternoon. However, she keeps herself preoccupied with many safety signals (e.g., Internet, television, radio, phone).

Felicia's fear of abandonment is starting to resemble agoraphobic tendencies. For example, she is reluctant to go to unfamiliar places (a restaurant, a party) and refuses to venture far from home. As a result, she misses out on sporting events and dreads the thought of attending sleepaway camp. Her chief safety signals are her parents, home, best friend, school nurse, track coach, and bronchial inhaler.

Data Check

Data from both the SAAS-C and SAAS-P suggested that Felicia's separation anxiety contained both FBA and FAb dimensions and was largely maintained by FPI. Data from the CASI, RCMAS, and MASC confirmed Felicia's strong fear of physical illness. She also reported mild worry and social anxiety. Most of her worries, however, emphasized her fear of physical illness (i.e., vomiting, trouble breathing) when she was alone or away from home, and were usually triggered by somatic sensations (e.g., upset stomach, difficulty breathing). The prescriptive treatment of choice was relaxation-based procedures. However, given her mild worries and social anxiety, she was also likely to benefit from cognitive-based procedures as well.

CHAPTER 4

Child Coping Skills I

It's Time to Relax

Who has time to relax? Between work and taking care of my children, I'm too tired to do anything else. My son won't even let me go to the bathroom by myself.

—CONCERNED PARENT

THE IMPORTANCE OF RELAXATION

When was the last time you set aside *quality* time for yourself? Did you feel guilty? Too frequently we are consumed by work, family, social, and community obligations. It doesn't help that youngsters have adopted our hurried lifestyles (Elkind, 2001). At the end of the day, an exhausted parent dreams of long hours of uninterrupted sleep, only to awaken to complaints of aches and pains and a pair of hypervigilant eyes staring at them in the middle of the night. A youngster's separation anxiety can become a parent's nightmare. We need to teach youngsters to help themselves by learning the value of relaxation.

Uncomfortable physical feelings comprise a big part of a youngster's separation anxiety. These physical feelings may occur randomly but are more typically triggered in response to anticipation of being alone or abandoned. For the young child (ages 3–7 years), the physical feelings themselves are anxiety provoking and trigger attachment behaviors (i.e., need for close proximity to caregivers) or dependence on safety signals.

For older children (ages 8–12 years) and adolescents, the physical feelings (e.g., scratchy throat, upset stomach) may trigger anticipation of dreaded outcomes (e.g., choking, getting sick). In this case, the fear of physical illness is worse than any actual symptoms. Typically, the dreaded outcomes have never occurred, and if so, only on rare occasions (e.g., stomach virus). During this developmental span, the physical feelings may be limited to one or two symptoms. Overall, the presence of uncomfortable physical feelings, no matter what their function, diminish a youngster's sense of personal control and augment the feeling of separation anxiety. Relation-based procedures can restore that control and diminish or eliminate the separation anxiety.

GOALS OF RELAXATION-BASED PROCEDURES

Naturally, one of the goals of relaxation-based procedures is to help children and adolescents manage the physical feelings in their bodies. For young children who may not yet be able to verbalize their separation-related worries, relaxation procedures can be employed as a first step toward helping them cope. For older children and adolescents, relaxation procedures may be applied in a prescriptive fashion based on their individual needs.

Relaxation-based procedures can also be employed as a means of reducing generalized anxiety and tension—which is especially important when working with separation-anxious youth, given the frequent co-occurrence of GAD (Kendall et al., 2001; Masi et al., 1999), behavioral inhibition, and difficult temperamental features (Kagan, 1994, 1997). As a general anxiety management strategy, relaxation-based procedures can help deactivate the cycle of anxious apprehension (Barlow, 2002; Eisen & Kearney, 1995). As a result, youngsters may become less easily frustrated and overwhelmed in their day-to-day activities. This improvement is an important first step, because youngsters need to develop strengths in order to confront, eventually, their fear-inducing scenarios.

The most fundamental step is to empower children to use relaxation-based procedures as a coping skill during separation-related situations. This step can be accomplished in two ways. First, teach youngsters to use relaxation-based procedures instead of avoidance behavior or safety signals to manage the physical sensations associated with separation-related situations. Second, teach parents to allow their child to use the relaxation-based procedures instead of relying on unhealthy parental maintenance factors. Loving parents do the best they can to *take away* a youngster's separation anxiety. Typical responses include overprotection (i.e., allowing the child to avoid separation-related events), reassurance, and if all else fails, coercive methods to terminate both the youngster's distress as well as their own (see Chapter 6 for a full discussion of parenting traps). Relaxation as a coping skill helps restore a youngster's sense of personal control and provides him or her with the ability to cope successfully with separation anxiety.

BASIC TOOLS AND PROCEDURES

In this section we discuss, demonstrate, and implement methods of progressive relaxation, diaphragmatic breathing, and visualization with Felicia (introduced in the Part III introduction). We also discuss modifications to these procedures in light of developmental concerns or comorbid problems.

Progressive Relaxation

You cannot be tense and relaxed at the same time (Jacobsen, 1974; Wolpe, 1992). Hence, progressive relaxation exercises involve first tensing different muscle groups, then releasing that tension and feeling the deep relaxation. The child or adolescent is taught to notice the difference between the uncomfortable feeling of tension and the pleasant feeling of deeply relaxed muscles. The tensing part is a constructive way (rather than crying or throwing temper tantrums) of dealing with tension and anxiety. The relaxation part helps to restore personal control and a general feeling of calmness in separation-anxiety-related scenarios.

Progressive relaxation is also associated with decrements in blood pressure, pulse, and respiration rates (Bernstein, Borkovec, & Hazlett-Stevens, 2000). More importantly, these exercises are ideal even for young children because they are simple. Progressive relaxation has been shown to reduce separation anxiety in children and adolescents as part of an integrated treatment program (Eisen et al., 2003; Eisen & Silverman, 1993, 1998; Kendall, 1994; Kendall et al., 1997). In Dialogue 4.1, we present the rationale for progressive relaxation exercises in the context of discussing Felicia's FAb. This excerpt is from the first treatment session and is appropriate for older children (at least 8 years) and adolescents.

Dialogue 4.1.

THERAPIST: Last week we discussed your fear of being alone and feeling uncomfortable in unfamiliar places.

FELICIA: (*Nods.*)

THERAPIST: We also talked about the physical feelings you experience when you're anxious, such as stomachaches, scratchy throat, and difficulty breathing. Did you have any of these feelings this week?

FELICIA: (*Nods.*)

THERAPIST: Can you tell me about them?

FELICIA: (*Sighs.*) A friend asked me to go with her to a Mexican restaurant.

THERAPIST: Did you go?

FELICIA: No . . . (*soft voice*).

THERAPIST: Why not?

FELICIA: I didn't feel well that night.

THERAPIST: Was it your stomach?

FELICIA: *Yes.* I didn't want to throw up in the restaurant.

THERAPIST: Has that ever happened?

FELICIA: No . . . but it could.

THERAPIST: Remember I told you that the only way to *overcome* anxiety is to *experience* anxiety?

FELICIA: (*Nods.*) You *want* me to go to the restaurant.

THERAPIST: Yes . . . but not right away. Going to the restaurant will show you that nothing bad will happen, and when you know that, your anxiety will lessen.

FELICIA: (*Shrugs.*) I don't know . . .

THERAPIST: Could you go with your parents?

FELICIA: I guess so . . .

THERAPIST: Felicia, I *want* you to be able to go to the restaurant, stay home alone, and run on the track team. But I also want you to be able to do these things *without* the fear, discomfort, or need for your parents to be present. Today, I'd like to teach you some progressive relaxation exercises. The idea is for you to first tense different parts of your body. For example, I'll ask you to hold out your hands and make fists—and when you're making these fists, squeeze really hard. Channel all the tension, frustration, and anxiety into your hands and arms. (*Demonstrates the exercise and cues Felicia to try.*)

FELICIA: (*Squeezes her fists.*)

THERAPIST: Good. When you get upset over little things or experience uncomfortable physical sensations, your body is telling you that it's overwhelmed. The *tensing* part of these exercises will help you get rid of a lot of your generalized anxiety and tension. If you practice regularly, you'll feel calmer, cooler, and more relaxed.

The next step in progressive relaxation is to *relax* those different parts of your body that you just tensed. First you tense (*squeezes fists*), and then you relax (*opens hands, loosens fingers*). It's important to notice the difference between the tension and the relaxation. You cannot be tense and relaxed at the same time. If *you* can make yourself tense, *you* can make yourself relaxed. (*Demonstrates the different muscle groups that will be utilized.*) Are you ready to practice?

FELICIA: Yes.

THERAPIST: Good.

General Considerations

Progressive relaxation exercises should be practiced sitting in a comfortable chair (e.g., a recliner) or lying on a couch or bed. Ideally, we recommend that youngsters close their eyes during the exercises as well as to practice in a dim setting. By doing so, they are more likely to experience another state and achieve the fullest feeling of relaxation. Of course, practicing in the dark may cause some discomfort, especially if a youngster fears being alone at night, has difficulty sitting or lying still, or has a limited attention span. If any discomfort is expressed, simply omit that part of the relaxation script (see Handout 1).

A second point to keep in mind concerns the timing intervals for the *tensing* and *relaxing* of the muscle groups. We generally recommend tensing from 3 to 5 seconds and relaxing for 5 seconds. Most youngsters can tolerate these intervals. Again, based on a youngster's age, temperamental intensity, and attention span, you may have to modify one or both of these intervals. For example, temperamentally intense youngsters such as Brian can tense their muscles for longer periods. However, the relaxation part may prove difficult and be perceived as boring. Youngsters with a limited attention span (ages 3–7 years), significant distractibility, or comorbid ADHD will have difficulty relaxing. In addition, youngsters with a comorbid GAD may have difficulty *letting go* due to a perceived loss of control. As a result, in these cases, you may want to focus more on the tensing, with briefer intervals (i.e., 1–3 seconds) of relaxation.

In addition to the timing intervals for these exercises, you should also pay careful attention to the intensity with which these exercises are performed. For example, some temperamentally intense youngsters may tighten their muscles so hard that they are at risk of hurting themselves (e.g., muscle cramping, chipping a tooth). The tensing part of the exercises should promote a feeling of mild discomfort that will soon be contrasted with maximal relaxation. Take some time to determine how each youngster responds to the various exercises to create meaningful and individualized relaxation regimens.

Creating a Mindset for Relaxation

In our view, progressive relaxation is not just about tensing and relaxing. It's about arming youngsters with a tool that empowers them to cope with separation anxiety and related problems. Rarely will you work with a youngster who struggles only with separation anxiety. At the very least, you will also need to address temperamental features. Some of the biggest barriers to treatment success include overcautiousness, low frustration tolerance, and a strong-willed nature. Getting a youngster to cooperate with the treatment program can become one big power struggle. For this reason, our treatment approach addresses both separation anxiety and oppositional behaviors. We view these behaviors as inextricably connected, especially in the context of an exposure-based program. As a result, our progressive relaxation script (Handout 1) contains exercises that address oppositional behaviors, if needed.

As you get ready to begin the relaxation part of the program, keep in mind that under normal circumstances, you will meet with the child or adolescent once per week. Many of the important events that occur during treatment will take place *in between* sessions. For this reason, we recommend making an audiotape/compact disc of the relaxation exercises (see page 62). In this way, youngsters can practice the exercises as a general anxiety management tool. More importantly, however, you can personalize the tape by talking and coaching them through the exercises.

Progressive Relaxation Script

In this section, we take you through the progressive relaxation script (adapted with permission from Ollendick & Cerny, 1981) one exercise at a time. We provide comments to help you understand the mindset, developmental nature, and best application of the exercises. In addition, we suggest helpful things to say that address contraindications (e.g., behavioral inhibition, low frustration tolerance, limited attention span) that may affect the successful implementation of the exercises. The complete script (see Handout 1 in Appendix II) is intended for older children (at least 9 years old) and adolescents who have an adequate attention span and minimal comorbidity. Later in the chapter we recommend a prescribed sequence of exercises based on developmental considerations. It's important to keep in mind that these exercises can be employed with children and adolescents experiencing a range of anxiety and related disorders.

1. THE INTRODUCTION

Okay, [insert child's name], it's time to relax. Close your eyes. Just loosen up all the muscles in your body. Anything that you're thinking about . . . school, family, or friends . . . just push those thoughts away. *This is your time.* Just relax. I want you to listen to the sound of my voice and perform the following exercises. Let's begin . . .

Comment

The introduction clearly sets the stage. We're encouraging the youngster to push his or her thoughts away and learn to focus on the relaxation. For most children and adolescents, this is no easy task and may seem completely unfamiliar. Youngsters with separation anxiety and related problems are used to fretting about school, family, and friends. Through practice, the child can learn to block out anxiety-provoking thoughts and focus on relaxation. Most importantly, however, we emphasize that *"this is your time"*—for the hurried and overwhelmed child, relaxation represents refuge. We want youngsters to look forward to relaxation and to practice regularly.

2. FISTS

[Insert child's name], this exercise is for your hands and fingers. First, hold your arms out in front of you. Now, make fists with both hands. Squeeze hard. All the tension, all the frustration, all the anxiety—hold it tight in your fists . . . Now relax . . . Open up your hands and let your fingers be loose. Notice the difference, [insert child's name], when your hands are all tight and tense, and when they are nice . . . and loose . . . and relaxed. That's how we want you to feel. Nice . . . and loose . . . and relaxed. Let's try this again . . . First, hold your arms out in front of you. Now, make fists with both hands. Clench your fists hard. Hold them . . . good. Now relax again . . . Just kind of settle down, get comfortable, and relax. You feel good . . . and warm . . . and lazy.

Helpful Things to Say

As we mentioned previously, some youngsters will have difficulty relaxing or letting go. This difficulty may stem from an inability to sit still or focus, or a perceived loss of control. If a youngster is fidgeting after the fists exercise, and is at least 8 years old, consider adding one or both of these sections to the script:

[Insert child's name], sometimes it's hard to relax. We may be thinking about other things, like school, family, or friends. If you are having trouble relaxing, just do the best you can to push those thoughts away. The more you practice, the easier it will be to relax.

[Insert child's name], sometimes . . . we are afraid to let go. If we let go, we think we might lose control. Actually, if you let go and allow the relaxation to sink in, you will be in *total control* and you will see how wonderful it feels to be relaxed.

3. BICEPS

The next exercise is for your hands and arms. First, hold your arms out to the side. Now, hold your arms up high and show me your muscles. Tense your biceps. Hold them . . . Show me how strong you are . . . much stronger than all the tension and anxiety. Good . . . Now let go and relax . . . Let your arms be loose and feel how nice that is. It feels good to relax . . . Let's try this again. First, hold your arms out to the side. Now, hold your arms up high and show me your muscles. Tense your biceps. Tighter . . . Good . . . Now relax . . . Notice the difference when your arms are all tight and tense, and when they are nice and loose and relaxed. That's how we want your arms to feel. Nice . . . and loose . . . and relaxed. You feel good, and warm, and lazy.

4. SHOULDERS AND BACK

The next exercise is for your shoulders. Tense your shoulders. Push them down. Try to touch the ground. Hold in tight . . . Good . . . Now relax . . . Just loosen up your shoulders and bring them back to their natural, comfortable position. That feels so much better. Let's try this again. Tense your shoulders. Push them down. Tighter . . . Great. Now relax . . . *It feels so good to let go.* Notice that when you relax your shoulders, your back relaxes too, and that feels good . . . Just try to relax your whole body. Let yourself get as loose as you can.

Helpful Things to Say

Many youngsters experiencing anxiety disorders have perfectionistic tendencies (see Chapter 5). Anything less than flawless performance is unacceptable. When you combine this need for perfection with a behaviorally inhibited temperament, low frustration tolerance is often the result. If you're working with a youngster who is at least 8 years old and has low frustration tolerance, consider adding this section to the script.

[Insert child's name], you don't have to shoulder the burdens of the world. You just have to do the best that you can. Sometimes we focus too much on our performance. It's easy to feel good about yourself when you are successful, like winning a game or getting a good grade. The hard part is feeling good even when things do not go your way. If you focus on your efforts, you can always feel good, no matter what the outcome. *Take the pressure off.* Just do the best that you can. Remember, [insert child's name], you cannot fail at anything if you keep trying. So focus on your efforts, keep trying, and do your best. This is what I want you to think about when you're tensing your shoulders.

5. MOUTH

[Insert child's name], sometimes when we feel tight and tense, we feel it in the mouth, the jaw, or the teeth. If you feel that way, here is an exercise to practice. Press your lips together. Press them hard. Hold them . . . Good. Now relax. *Just let your mouth be loose. It feels so good to let go.* Let's try this again. Press your lips together. Press hard. Hold them . . . Good. Now relax again. *Just let your mouth be loose.* That feels so much better.

6. FOREHEAD

The next exercise is for your forehead. Make wrinkles on your forehead. *Raise your eyebrows.* All the tension, all the frustration, all the anxiety—hold it all in your forehead. Now relax . . . Let your forehead be smooth. Your forehead feels nice and smooth and relaxed. Let's try this again. Make wrinkles on your forehead. *Raise your eyebrows.* Hold them tight until I count to three. One . . . Two . . . Three . . . Now let it all go. No wrinkles anywhere. Your face feels nice and smooth and relaxed.

Comment

For children 4–8 years old, consider substituting the forehead exercise with the following *Mean Face* exercise. This exercise is especially helpful for temperamentally intense, strong-willed youngsters whose low frustration tolerance often gets the best of them.

7. MEAN FACE

The next exercise is for your whole face. Scrunch up your face—make wrinkles on your forehead. Raise your eyebrows. Push out your lower jaw.

Frown big. *Make a mean face.* Hold it all tight . . . Now relax . . . No more wrinkles. Your face feels nice and smooth and relaxed.

Why did I ask you to make a mean face? Sometimes when we get angry, we say mean things, hurtful things, to the people we care about, like, *I hate you* or *I will never play with you again.* Sometimes we *do* mean things, like pushing people or throwing things when we get upset. [Insert child's name], it would be better to make a *mean face.* No consequences for that. It's a great way of getting rid of your anger.

Let's try it again. *Show me your mean face.* Hold it tight . . . Good. Now relax . . . No wrinkles anywhere. Your face feels nice and smooth and relaxed.

8. STOMACH

The next exercise is for your stomach. Tighten up your stomach. Hold it. Don't move . . . Now relax. Just kind of settle down, get comfortable, and relax. Let your stomach come back out where it belongs. That feels so much better. Let's try this again. Tighten up . . . Tighten hard . . . Hold it. Now relax. [Insert child's name], notice the difference between a tight stomach and a relaxed one. That's how we want your stomach to feel. Nice . . . and loose . . . and relaxed. Now you can relax completely.

Comment

The stomach exercise is especially helpful for children and adolescents who have a strong fear of physical illness. Any time a youngster feels queasy in the stomach (e.g., fears vomiting), he or she can practice this exercise. It will help restore a sense of control.

The stomach exercise is the last progressive relaxation exercise in the script. For older children (at least 10 years old) and adolescents who have a good attention span, consider adding the following summary.

9. SUMMARY OF EXERCISES

[Insert child's name], let's make sure that all your muscles are nice and loose and relaxed. Your stomach should be resting in its natural, comfortable position. Your whole face is completely smooth. No wrinkles anywhere. No tension in your mouth. No tension in your shoulders. And remember, [insert child's name], you don't have to shoulder the burdens of the world. Just do the best you can. Your hands and arms feel loose and relaxed and your fingers may feel a bit tingly.

Comment

Based on our experience, most youngsters respond favorably to this sequence of progressive relaxation exercises. Of course, you can personalize the script by adding (e.g., chest, legs, feet) or eliminating specific muscle groups based on a youngster's specific somatic complaints.

Diaphragmatic Breathing

Most people take breathing for granted—until, of course, it becomes irregular. In general, a fear of suffocation is often associated with anxiety and panic (Asmundson & Stein, 1994; Eisen, Rapee, & Barlow, 1990; McNally & Eke, 1996). Specifically, carbon dioxide hypersensitivity, a characteristic often associated with adult panic disorder (e.g., Papp, Klein, & Gorman, 1993; Perna, Bertani, Arancio, Ronchi, & Bellodi, 1995), has been demonstrated in children with separation anxiety (Pine et al., 2000). In addition, childhood respiratory illness (e.g., asthma) is often linked with adult panic disorder (Perna, Bertani, Politi, Columbo, & Bellodi, 1997; Verburg, Griez, Meijer, & Pols, 1995). Hence, a heightened sensitivity to somatic sensations (prompting a fear of physical illness) in the context of separation anxiety may set the stage for the development of adolescent and adult panic.

Breathing exercises are one of the easiest ways to elicit the relaxation response (Benson & Stuart, 1992) and have been shown to be effective in reducing anxiety, panic, muscle tension, and headaches. In our experience, diaphragmatic breathing is a simple and natural way to help youngsters manage physical sensations and restore feelings of personal control. Breathing exercises can be used as part of a general anxiety or anger management program, as a coping tool in separation-anxiety-related scenarios, or with youngsters who specifically fear suffocation. In Dialogue 4.2, we model and practice diaphragmatic breathing exercises with Felicia.

Dialogue 4.2.

THERAPIST: When you feel tightness in your chest, do you breathe through your mouth?

FELICIA: (*Nods.*)

THERAPIST: When you breathe in through your mouth, your breathing may become shallow, irregular, or rapid. You may feel like you're losing control and unable to catch your breath.

FELICIA: (*Nods, then sighs.*)

THERAPIST: When that happens, breathe in deeply through your nose, and then breathe out through your mouth. (*Demonstrates.*) As you fill your lungs with air, breathing becomes easier. As you realize that you do have some control over your breathing, you will feel more in control. Let's practice. Let me see you breathe in . . .

FELICIA: (*Breathes in too forcefully.*)

THERAPIST: Watch me. (*Breathes in slowly, effortlessly, and deeply.*)

FELICIA: (*Breathes in slowly and deeply.*)

THERAPIST: Good . . . Now watch me breathe out. (*Breathes in . . . breathes out in a gentle stream of air.*) When you breathe out, I want you to gently blow all the tension a mile away.

General Considerations

Be sure to demonstrate the proper form, timing, and intensity of the breathing exercises. For example, some youngsters may breathe in and out through their mouth. As a result, their breathing may be too shallow or rapid and could lead to hyperventilation when they are under stress. We recommend that youngsters breathe in through their nose and breathe out through their mouth in 3-second intervals. Some temperamentally intense youngsters may breathe in and out too quickly or may hold their breath for longer intervals. In both cases, breathing this way may increase the youngster's anxiety.

The intensity of a youngster's breathing is another factor to consider. For example, some youngsters may breathe too forcefully. Be sure to demonstrate how to breathe in slowly, gradually filling your lungs with air. As you breathe out, do so by gently blowing a stream of air. Hold your hand out in front of your face and show the youngster how you feel the gentle air against your palm. Have the child practice until he or she feels the sensation of a gentle breeze.

Adding Breathing Exercises to the Script

For older children and adolescents with a good attention span, the breathing exercises can follow the last progressive relaxation exercise (i.e., stomach) or the summary of the exercises. Our script includes a transition to keep the flow of the exercises smooth. We modify the script for younger children accordingly (see "Developmental Considerations," p. 61).

[Insert child's name], now it's time to practice our breathing exercises. Most people don't know how to breathe to relax. The trick is to first breathe in deeply through your nose. As you breathe in, be sure to fill up your lungs with air and hold that breath until I tell you to breathe out. When I tell you to breathe out, pretend that you are the wind, and blow that tension a mile away. When you breathe in, you breathe in the good energy, and when you breathe out, you let go of your fear. Let's practice. Try to stick to my pace.

Let me *see* you breathe in . . . Let me *hear* you breathe out . . . Let me *see* you breathe in . . . Let me *hear* you breathe out. And as you breathe out, pretend that you are the wind, and blow all that tension a mile away. [Repeat.]

Comment

When a youngster breathes in, you want to see him or her fill the chest with air. When he or she breathes out, you want to hear the sound of the wind. This exercise ties in nicely with the visualization exercises described next.

Visualization

In order to render the breathing exercises more salient, we recommend using visualization exercises. The image of traveling in a hot-air balloon (e.g., Ginsburg, Silverman, & Kurtines, 1995) fits our purpose nicely. The youngster's breathing supplies the balloon with air and takes him or her to a place that is safe and comfortable. You can personalize the image based on a youngster's favorite place (e.g., vacation spot) or you can simply use our script. In explaining the rationale for the visualization exercises, we reiterate the point that the only way to *overcome* anxiety is to *experience* anxiety. We make it clear that *physically* escaping from the separation-anxiety encounter is not ideal. Rather, *mentally* escaping—that is, taking him- or herself to another place—can be helpful during the stress-inducing exposures.

Adding Visualization to the Script

For older children and adolescents with a good attention span, consider adding one or both brief visualization scenarios to the script. As you can see, we combine each of the scenes with the breathing exercises to capture the full effect. The script begins with a transition.

[Insert child's name], I want you to keep breathing in through your nose and breathing out through your mouth. At the same time, I want you to pretend that you are stepping aboard a hot-air balloon. As you breathe in and breathe out, you will fill the hot air balloon, and it will take you wherever you would like to go.

SCENE 1

Suddenly, you find yourself high in the sky . . . It's a beautiful spring day . . . The sky is blue . . . You feel the warmth of the sun shining against your forehead . . . A cool breeze blows by [make a gentle swooshing sound] . . . You look down below and see the magnificent forest . . . This is where you go when *you need to relax.*

Let me *see you* breathe in . . . Let me *hear you* breathe out . . .

Let me *see you* breathe in . . . Let me *hear you* breathe out.

And as you breathe out, pretend you are the wind and blow the tension a mile away.

SCENE 2

The hot-air balloon lands on the beach. As you step down, you feel the hot sand against your toes. You see the children swimming in the ocean. The seagulls are flying above you. Just stand there, [insert child's name], and breathe in the ocean air. This is where you go when *you need to relax.*

Let me *see you* breathe in . . . Let me *hear you* breathe out . . .

Let me *see you* breathe in . . . Let me *hear you* breathe out . . .

And as you breathe out, pretend you are the wind and blow the tension a mile away.

Comment

The visualization scenes are the last relaxation tools in the script. For older children and adolescents with a good attention span and minimal comorbidity, the visualization scenes enhance the degree of relaxation experienced. In addition, the scenes give greater meaning to the breathing exercises. Use your judgment in deciding whether a particular child may benefit from the scenes or may be unable to tolerate the added length of the script. We recommend ending the script with a personalized conclusion.

SCRIPT CONCLUSION

Try to stay as relaxed as you can. All your muscles should be nice and loose and relaxed. I want you to listen to this tape every night before you go to bed. You may even fall asleep before the tape is finished. If you listen every night, you will sleep better. You will be calmer. The little things will not bother you as much. But the real trick, [insert child's name], is that I want you to use these exercises in the situations that make you feel scared, like [insert relevant scenarios]. And all you have to do is try your best. And you know what you are going to realize really soon . . . *There is nothing that you cannot do.*

Developmental Considerations

Consider the following script modifications based on age and attention span. These modifications are designed to ensure that each youngster benefits from the relaxation script and to increase the likelihood of regular practice.

Ages 3–4

Keep the exercises simple and concrete and limit yourself to the use of two or three key ones. Emphasize relaxation as a coping skill in specific separation-anxiety scenarios. The idea is to encourage the child to practice the exercises instead of crying, whining, throwing a temper tantrum, or avoiding specific situations (e.g., being alone, sleeping alone). To make practicing the exercises salient, consider the use of tangible contingent rewards (see Chapter 7). Consider modifying the exercises as follows:

BREATHING EXERCISES

Smell the roses [breathe in] . . . Blow out the candles [breathe out] . . . [Repeat.]

PROGRESSIVE RELAXATION EXERCISES

Stomach

Make your stomach tight . . . Squeeze hard . . . Let go . . . [Repeat.]

Fists

Show me your fists . . . Squeeze tight . . . Let go . . . [Repeat.]

Ages 5–9

For most youngsters in this age category, the entire script is too long. Some 8-year-olds with a good attention span, however, can tolerate and benefit from the entire script. In general, you should stick to the basic sequence of the script, with some suggested omissions as follows:

Include	*Omit*
Introduction	Helpful things to say
Fists	Summary of exercises
Biceps	Visualization
Mouth	
Mean face	
Stomach	
Breathing	
Conclusion	

Ages 10 Years and Older

In general, the majority of children and adolescents in this age category can benefit from the entire relaxation script. Of course, there is room to individualize for specific youngsters, based on their attention span, temperamental intensity, and comorbidity. Use your judgment to determine which (if any) helpful things to say or visualization scenes are worthwhile to incorporate.

Preparing and Recording the Relaxation Tape

First, fully familiarize yourself with the entire script. Second, determine the specific set of exercises to be utilized, based on the youngster's age, attention span, temperamental intensity, and comorbidity. Third, spend part of a session demonstrating the specific exercises to the youngster. Model the proper form and intensity, then have the youngster practice until he or she performs the exercises on cue (e.g., "Show me the fists"). During this session, you will be able to evaluate the extent of the exercises a youngster can tolerate.

Consider recording a practice tape to help you regulate the tone and pitch of the tension and relaxation segments of the exercises. The next step is to decide *when* you will record the tape. Ideally, we recommend recording the tape as you perform the script with the child or adolescent. Be sure to encourage youngsters to *perform* the exercises rather than simply closing their eyes and relaxing. In some cases, you may have to *record and demonstrate* the exercises simultaneously to keep the youngster on task. Most of the time, however, you may need to periodically check to make sure the exercises are being performed. Consider using a hand signal to help the youngster stay on track.

Alternatively, if a youngster becomes easily distracted or has difficulty sitting still, consider recording the tape prior to the session. Five- and 6-year-olds may become too distracted or act silly during the recording. You can introduce the exercises during a session, record the tape later, then practice the exercises, using the tape, the following visit. No need to make a tape for children younger than 5 years. Simply emphasize practicing the exercises in separation-anxiety scenarios.

Practicing Relaxation

Although the relaxation script can be used at any time, we recommend that the child or adolescent practice at night shortly before bedtime. The script is designed so that the first part (progressive relaxation) is the most active, followed by the more tranquil breathing and visualization parts. As a result, many youngsters will fall asleep before the script concludes. Keep in mind, however, that some youngsters may become too stimulated by the exercises and have difficulty falling asleep. If this occurs, determine a feasible time to practice during the day (e.g., before or after school). Regular practice serves as a general anxiety management strategy. Consistent practice will help diminish a youngster's general anxiety and tension. More importantly, however, the youngster can benefit from the power of the exercises during in vivo separation-anxiety-related exposures.

To cultivate relaxation as a coping skill, demonstrate how to perform each of the exercises (without the tape) in an unobtrusive way. Consider our suggestions for disguising the progressive relaxation and breathing exercises:

- *Fists*: Cross arms and tuck fists in underarms.
- *Biceps*: Extend arms and hold close to side.
- *Shoulders*: Same as script.
- *Mouth*: Keep closed.
- *Forehead*: Raise eyebrows.
- *Mean face*: Face the wall.
- *Stomach*: Same as script.
- Breathe in deeply through the nose for 3 seconds and breathe out through the mouth for 3 seconds without making the swooshing sound.

Clinical Tip

Encourage youngsters to choose three of their favorite progressive relaxation exercises. Demonstrate how you count to yourself (i.e., 1 ... 2 ... 3 ...) during the tension and relaxation segments of the exercises. In addition, demonstrate how to combine several of the exercises at a time to help manage overwhelming sensations of anxiety or frustration. Counting is also helpful during the breathing exercises as well.

Homework

Encourage youngsters to practice the exercises (i.e., listen to the tape) once per day and to try the exercises (without the tape) in separation-anxiety scenarios that naturally occur during the week. In Chapter 3 we introduced the "What's Happening to Me?" DD to help you determine whether separation anxiety was maintained by bodily symptoms, anxious cognitions, or both. Once treatment begins and it becomes clear that a youngster is prone to somatic symptoms, replace the DD with our "Coping with My Body" record (see Handout 4 in Appendix II). This measure helps youngsters keep track of bodily feelings, their impact, as well as the relaxation exercises they utilized to help them cope.

WHAT'S NEXT?

On the following pages we present step-by-step guidelines for teaching and practicing cognitive self-control, cognitive therapy, and problem-solving exercises with separation-anxious children and adolescents. We also introduce our third case example, a 10-year-old African American girl, Natalie, who is afraid of being abandoned by her mother, Mrs. C. Natalie lives with her parents and younger brother. She is afraid to be dropped off at birthday parties, play dates, sleep-overs, or after-school activities (e.g., soccer, dance). In fact, she refuses to participate unless her mother stays with her the entire time. Familiar places such as school are not problematic, as long as her mother promises to pick her up on time. If her mother is a few minutes late, however, Natalie becomes frantic, paces back and forth, cries, and demands that the nurse call her mother's cell phone. When Natalie's mother needs to run errands, walk the dog, or visit with a neighbor, being left with her father and brother is not enough to quell her anxiety.

Data Check

Data from both the SAAS-C and SAAS-P suggested that Natalie's separation anxiety was primarily comprised of a fear of abandonment and maintained by worry about calamitous events (WCE) to herself and mother. Data from the RCMAS and MASC confirmed Natalie's worried/oversensitive nature. Her chief safety signals included her mother's presence (in person and over the phone), and promises to stay at home or to pick her up on time. The prescriptive treatment of choice is cognitive-based procedures.

CHAPTER 5

Child Coping Skills II

You Are What You Think

> What if she [mom] forgets to pick me up? What if she gets in a car accident? *Where is she?* (*Looking at watch*) Mom ... (*Starts to cry, runs into the school building.*)
>
> —NATALIE

THE PERILS OF WORRY

Life is full of worry. How many times have you laid in bed at night, unable to sleep because your worries about work, family, finances, or the state of the world simply refused to take a rest? Imagine if you heard a noise outside your window at night. Could you ignore it? Was it just the wind? Think of what your life would be like if frequent and intense thoughts about your personal safety and that of others kept popping into your head ... if your ability to suppress them was limited, and if you really believed them. Welcome to the mind of the separation-anxious youngster.

The Nature of Worry

Worry can be broadly defined as apprehensive expectation in the absence of realistically dangerous outcomes (Barlow, 2002; Borkovec, Robinson, Pruzinsky, & DePree, 1983). Sometimes it's hard to believe that children worry. After all, childhood *should be* a relatively carefree period. Childhood worry is indeed a normative phenomenon.

65

Some 70% of primary school children reported at least one worry (Muris, Meesters, Merckelbach, Sermon, & Zwakhalen, 1998; Muris, Merckelbach, Gadet, & Moulaert, 2000; Silverman et al., 1995). This type of worry should be distinguished from clinical worry (i.e., excessive and uncontrollable), which occurs in about 5% of youngsters (Muris, Merckelbach, Meesters, & van den Brand, 2002). Frequent and intense worries about the personal safety of self and others are characteristic of SAD. Clinical levels of worry are also prominent across DSM-IV anxiety disorders (generalized and social anxiety disorders, panic, and specific phobias).

When it comes to worrying, we are not all created equal. The "ability" to worry requires anticipating future events as well as pondering many possible (catastrophic) outcomes (Vasey, Crnic, & Carter, 1994). These abilities tend to emerge around 7 years of age and become crystallized during middle childhood (Piaget, 1970; Vasey et al., 1994). Recent data suggest that worrisome thoughts are more likely to become prominent in older children (at least age 8; Muris et al., 2000) and are associated with increased age and cognitive development (Muris et al., 2002). Thus, young children (ages 6 and under) may not fully appreciate the realistic likelihood and actual impact of anxious events (Izard, 1994; Nelles & Barlow, 1988; Piacentini & Bergman, 2001). As a result, they are not in the best position to cope with their anxiety (Bogels & Zigterman, 2000).

Functions of Worry

Why worry? Let's take a moment to examine the functions of worry in relation to anxiety, in general, and separation anxiety, in particular. In this way, you will be in the best position to help separation-anxious youngsters cope with their worry.

It's important to keep in mind that some youngsters may be reluctant to *give up* their worries. For example, worry may be perceived as a positive way of dealing with anticipatory threat (Borkovec & Roemer, 1995; Cartwright-Hatton & Wells, 1997). The separation-anxious youngster may become hypervigilant—that is, *ready for anything*—if worried about being alone or abandoned. Thus, worry may facilitate coping and diminish feelings of uncontrollability (Craske, 1999). Keep in mind, however, that evidence fails to support this relationship (e.g., Borkovec, Hazlett-Stevens, & Diaz, 1999). In fact, worry appears more likely to serve as an avoidance tactic (Craske, 1999). So, the more the youngster worries, becomes hypervigilant, and *still does nothing*, the more aversive the separation-related scenarios may become.

We have found this relationship to be the case in our work. For example, in separation-anxious youth, elevated worry was associated with greater anxiety and resistance during exposures (Hahn et al., 2003). In other words, youngsters were less likely to "test out" their worries if they truly believed that calamitous events would occur. Thus, worrying is negatively reinforcing—that is, it provides relief by encouraging avoidance of unpleasant exposures. This is why cognitive-based procedures are so important in breaking the cycle of anxious apprehension.

Negative Self-Talk: What If the Glass Breaks?

We all talk to ourselves. Think of the last time you noticed someone talking to themselves *out loud*. It may have seemed a bit strange, depending upon the context of the situation. For youngsters, however, talking to themselves is completely natural, perhaps because they have a less developed ability to self-monitor their actions (Piacentini & Bergman, 2001). So, talking to oneself is fine. The *content* of one's self-talk is another story.

For example, the self-statements of anxious youth have a tendency to be negative, hostile, and catastrophic in content (Rietveld, Prins, & van Beest, 2002; Treadwell & Kendall, 1996). These patterns of faulty or negative thinking, referred to as cognitive distortions, may increase vulnerability to anxiety disorders (e.g., Beck, Emery, & Greenberg, 1985; Craske, 1999; Vasey & MacLeod, 2001). Studies have demonstrated that cognitive distortions are associated with anxiety and its disorders in children and adolescents (Bell-Dollan & Wessler, 1994; Epkins, 1996; Leitenberg, Yost, & Carroll-Wilson, 1986; Leung & Wong, 1998; Weems et al., 2000).

COGNITIVE DISTORTIONS AND COPING

Let's examine some of the central cognitive distortions that may undermine an anxious youngster's coping efforts and that have relevance for separation anxiety. These include misappraisals of danger, misperceptions of coping abilities, and a focus on failure (Kendall, 2000; Kendall & Chansky, 1991).

Misappraisals of Danger

The tendency here is to misinterpret ambiguous situations as threatening (Barrett, Rapee, Dadds, & Ryan, 1996; Bogels & Zitgerman, 2000; Chorpita, Albano, & Barlow, 1996). The separation-anxious youngster's thoughts may be frequently tainted with threats of danger and harm to self and others. In the extreme form, catastrophizing (i.e., expecting the worst) may occur. It's understandable for a youngster to panic and become hysterical if a parent's lateness is viewed to be the result of a fatal car accident.

Misperceptions of Coping Abilities

Overestimating potential sources of threat begins the cycle of anxious apprehension. Underestimating one's coping ability sets the stage for avoidance (Bogels & Zigterman, 2000). Why bother putting yourself in situations if you believe you cannot cope? The separation-anxious youngster is likely to take the safe way out by staying glued to a major caregiver or safety signal. These avoidance efforts further reinforce the perception of an inept coping ability and strengthen the separation-anxiety response.

Focus on Failure

Several specific cognitive distortions encourage self-evaluations that emphasize failure. These include:

- All-or-nothing thinking: Outcomes are evaluated as either perfect or a complete failure.
- Overgeneralization: A single negative event is made the basis for evaluating a variety of situations.
- Personalization: Responsibility for any negative outcome is self-attributed.
- Selective abstraction: Only the negative aspects of an event are emphasized.

Focusing on failure makes it less likely that one will initiate coping behaviors and persist in the face of anxiety (Bandura, 1988). The addition of specific temperamental features (e.g., behavioral inhibition, low frustration tolerance) may further weaken the separation-anxious youngster's perception of control.

GOALS OF COGNITIVE-BASED PROCEDURES

One of the goals of cognitive-based procedures is to teach children and adolescents to identify excessive and uncontrollable worries, negative self-talk, and distorted cognitions. An effective way to overcome anxiety is to first recognize how these self-defeating thought patterns inter-fere with psychosocial functioning. The second goal, of course, is to help youngsters develop more constructive ways of thinking. Working together, you help youngsters develop increasingly accurate ways of evaluating potential risk and danger in separation-anxiety-related sce-narios. By doing so, you foster perceptions of control and inspire the enactment of newly acquired coping efforts.

Given that the self-statements of anxious youth tend to be nega-tive, it would seem intuitive to help youngsters think in more positive ways. However, *eliminating* negative rather than increasing positive self-statements appears to be a more powerful tool in the anxious child's coping repertoire. Non-negative or *healthy thinking* (Kendall, 1992) has been consistently associated with positive treatment outcomes (e.g., Eisen & Silverman, 1993, 1998; Treadwell & Kendall, 1996). Healthy thinking inspires *coping self-talk*—that is, a constructive plan of action. Simply thinking in positive ways, at best, serves as a brief distraction.

DEVELOPMENTAL CONSIDERATIONS

Teaching youngsters healthy thinking strategies is one thing. Whether or not these strategies are retained and implemented is quite another. For any given youngster, your choice of cognitive therapy interventions will depend largely on developmental considerations. For example, young children have a less developed ability to identify and regulate their emotions (Izard, 1994). Even older children and adolescents may have difficulty verbalizing their worries and negative self-statements. Drawing cartoon strips with empty thought bubbles to be filled in by youngsters can help them identify both fearful and coping thoughts (Kendall, 1990; Silverman, 1989). A blackboard or easel is suitable for this purpose.

In addition, children and some adolescents may have limited abstract thinking abilities (Piaget, 1967), so the cognitive therapy strat-egies should be presented in basic, concrete terms. Sometimes, how-ever, being concrete is not enough. You may need to get creative in your efforts to help youngsters acquire the cognitive skills.

Getting Creative with Play Therapy

Play therapy applications can be easily integrated into a cognitive-behavioral framework for anxious youth (see Friedberg & McClure, 2002; Knell, 1993). A variety of strategies has been used with this popu-lation, including coping-oriented storytelling (Friedberg, 1994), puppet play (Friedberg, Friedberg, & Friedberg, 2001), rational games and coloring books (Waters, 1979, 1980), and making masks (Friedberg & McClure, 2002). These strategies are designed to facilitate Socratic-type dialogues and create a sense of mastery.

Several strategies have relevance for children with separation anxiety. For example, Lyness (1993) suggests that *repetition* of play activities (e.g., hide and seek) can help children master the fear of being alone. In addition, *identifying* with more powerful figures (e.g., superheros; Kendall, 1990) can help children feel safe when caregivers are absent as well as confident about their ability to keep intruders away.

The Future Is Now: The Importance of Exposure

Perhaps the biggest obstacle to conducting cognitive therapy interventions with youngsters is their "here-and-now" orientation (Piacentini & Bergman, 2001). Youngsters are more likely to live moment to moment. The future is too abstract. It's not real. Cognitive therapy strategies may make no sense in the absence of real-life experiences and applications. For this reason, cognitive procedures are rarely implemented without an exposure component. Exposures make the future immediate and give youngsters the opportunity to "reality test" their faulty beliefs.

It is widely recognized that exposures provide opportunities for anxiety reduction as well as for developing a sense of mastery (for reviews, see Albano & Kendall, 2002; Ollendick & King, 2002). Keep in mind, however, that the *evaluation* of the exposure assumes great importance. For example, sometimes the success of an exposure is not judged by whether or not the youngster navigated the separation anxious event but by the *degree of anxiety* experienced. Hence, the youngster may refuse to recognize or understand the importance of *experiencing anxiety*. As a result, exposures followed by *unhealthy* evaluations will help maintain separation anxiety.

Exposing children and adolescents to separation-related scenarios is one challenge (see Chapters 8–10). Helping them learn to evaluate outcomes constructively is another. The second challenge is addressed in this chapter.

BASIC TOOLS AND PROCEDURES

In this section, we discuss, demonstrate, and implement cognitive self-control (self-monitoring, self-evaluation, self-reinforcement), cognitive therapy, and problem-solving procedures with Natalie.

Cognitive Self-Control

Think of the last time you became frustrated or anxious. How long did it take before your emotions overwhelmed you? Was your response proportional to the demands of the situation? It's not so easy to regulate our emotions. Think of what it may be like for a youngster with a high-intensity temperament, low frustration tolerance, and a sensitivity to separation anxiety. Simply *thinking about* a caregiver's impending absence or not having access to a safety signal can trigger anxious apprehension that spirals out of hand.

For this reason, cognitive self-control training plays a fundamental role in our efforts to in help youngsters with separation anxiety manage their emotions. In self-control programs, youngsters are taught to identify distorted cognitions and to develop more constructive ways of thinking (e.g., Friedberg & McClure, 2002; Kendall, 2000).

Recognizing Separation Anxiety

The first step in helping children and adolescents to overcome separation anxiety is to increase their *awareness* of separation anxiety. This is no easy task. For reasons previously discussed, young children are less likely to be aware of their thoughts or feelings. Older children and adolescents may engage in cognitive or emotional avoidance (blocking thoughts or feelings) to minimize anxious apprehension (Young, 1990). Because avoidance on any level, not just behavioral (i.e., avoidance of separation-related scenarios), will strengthen anxiety, encouraging youngsters to self-monitor is worthwhile for several reasons.

First, because of a youngster's here-and-now orientation, once an anxiety-provoking event passes, it's almost like it doesn't exist. Any effort to discuss the event may be met with resistance. Self-monitoring is an excellent way of circumventing cognitive and emotional avoidance.

Second, limited memory capacities are likely to result in vague and nonspecific recollections of weekly separation-anxious events. As a result, your efforts to teach cognitive therapy exercises may be hampered. Daily self-monitoring not only facilitates accurate recording but also allows you to tailor cognitive interventions to a youngster's specific needs.

Finally, self-monitoring is an excellent way to gauge a youngster's motivation and commitment to your treatment program. Keep in mind that many youngsters will view this process as inconvenient or even a nuisance. Early efforts to address lost, forgotten, or incomplete daily diaries may improve later adherence and therapeutic outcome (Eisen &

Kearney, 1995). In Dialogue 5.1, we present the rationale for self-monitoring to Natalie (introduced at the end of Chapter 4).

Dialogue 5.1

THERAPIST: Natalie, you did a great job with your "What's Happening to Me?" diary. I noticed you reported mostly "what if?" thoughts.

NATALIE: (*Nods.*)

THERAPIST: I'd like to show you a new diary. It's called "Coping with My Worries." (*Gives it to Natalie.*)

NATALIE: (*Sour expression*) Do I have to *keep doing this*?

THERAPIST: I realize that keeping track of your worries is not much fun.

NATALIE: I don't want to think about it.

THERAPIST: I know . . . But remember, the only way you *overcome* anxiety is to *experience* anxiety. So I want you to think about your worries *even* if it makes you uncomfortable.

NATALIE: (*Sighs.*)

THERAPIST: Natalie, please take a look at the new diary. (*She complies.*) It's not just about your worries anymore. Look at the columns. (*Points to* "Coping Thoughts and Praise.") If you're willing to keep track of your worries, I can teach you good (healthy) ways to think so you can learn to cope with your anxiety.

NATALIE: Do I have to do this *every day*?

THERAPIST: I only see you once a week. All the important stuff happens outside of our sessions. Without the diaries, you would have to remember *everything*.

NATALIE: I can do that.

THERAPIST: (*Smiles.*) What did you have for lunch yesterday?

NATALIE: (*Giggles.*) A *sandwich*?

THERAPIST: What kind?

NATALIE: (*Pauses.*) I don't know . . .

THERAPIST: It's not so easy to remember. And if you don't want to *think* about your worries, you may forget just how anxious you were. Will you keep track of your thoughts?

NATALIE: *Yes.*

THERAPIST: Are you ready to learn how to cope with your anxiety?

NATALIE: (*Smiles, then nods her head.*)

THERAPIST: Great.

You Don't Have to Be Perfect

Remember, the outcome of an event is determined by how the person *evaluates* the event. It doesn't help that the separation-anxious youngster is living in a perfectionistic society. Parents, teachers, and coaches expect nothing less than the best from youngsters. Of course, most parents *tell* their children simply to "do their best." However, what most parents *show* their children by selectively attending to specific accomplishments (e.g., academics, sports) is another story. As a result, it may be difficult for a youngster to preserve self-esteem when his or her performance is below par.

To complicate matters, separation-anxious youngsters are particularly vulnerable to cognitive distortions that emphasize failure. For this reason, we are strong believers in teaching youngsters to evaluate outcomes based on *effort* and *partial successes* rather than performance (Kendall, 1990). In Dialogue 5.2, we use these concepts to help Natalie reevaluate a disastrous birthday party. To help you understand the context of the outcome, we provide some background information.

Prior to the beginning of treatment, Natalie had attended a birthday party with her mother. She had refused to get out of the car unless her mother promised to stay with her the entire time. Mrs C. agreed, and the two of them stood in the back of the room with Natalie glued to her side. After 5 minutes, Mrs. C. remembered that she needed some items from a nearby store in the shopping plaza. She insisted that Natalie remain at the party and that "she would be right back." Natalie became frantic, forcefully squeezed her mother's arm, and repeatedly screamed, "*You promised!*" Mrs. C. became frustrated, threatened punishment (i.e., removal of privileges), and immediately took her daughter home.

Dialogue 5.2

THERAPIST: Natalie, can you tell me about the party?

NATALIE: (*Gives stern look, rolls her eyes.*) It's over . . . I don't want to talk about it.

THERAPIST: When was the last time you went to a birthday party?

NATALIE: *That was the last time.*

THERAPIST: I meant *before* last weekend.

NATALIE: (*Pauses.*) I don't remember. What does it matter?

THERAPIST: It matters a great deal. You *were willing* to try. And *you did stay* for 5 minutes. Did you ever do that before?

NATALIE: I guess not.

THERAPIST: Natalie, you cannot fail at anything as long as you keep trying. The only time we fail is when we get frustrated, give up, and quit. And the worst part about quitting is that you never would have known that you could have accomplished your goal.

So, don't focus on the fact that you became anxious and left the party early [performance]. Think about your willingness to try [effort] and that you stayed for 5 minutes [partial success]. You don't have to be perfect.

NATALIE: My mom doesn't think so. She took away my TV for a week.

THERAPIST: I'll talk to her. (*Smiles.*) You just weren't ready to be left alone. Will you try going to another party?

NATALIE: I guess so.

THERAPIST: How will you evaluate how you do?

NATALIE: If I try hard.

THERAPIST: How long will you try to stay?

NATALIE: (*Pauses.*) *Ten minutes?*

THERAPIST: That's great. Let's focus on partial successes based on your efforts. This way, as long as you try, you will always be successful.

Never Put Yourself Down

Other people will do it for you. There will always be someone out there who evaluates your performance in an overly critical way. Who is this person for you? A boss? A colleague? A family member? If we don't evaluate ourselves in constructive ways, who will? Teaching youngsters to praise themselves based on their coping efforts is the most important part of self-control programs. Healthy doses of self-praise will preserve a youngster's self-esteem in the face of adversity. In Dialogue 5.3, we help Natalie understand the importance of self-praise.

Dialogue 5.3.

THERAPIST: Natalie, do you know what it means to praise someone?

NATALIE: (*Nods her head.*) You tell them they did good.

THERAPIST: That's right. Do your mom and dad always praise you?

NATALIE: (*Giggles.*)

THERAPIST: Do they get frustrated with your behavior sometimes?

NATALIE: (*Sighs, nods her head.*)

THERAPIST: How about your teachers?

NATALIE: (*Giggles again.*) They don't like it when I forget my homework.

THERAPIST: Do your friends always praise you?

NATALIE: I just had a fight with my best friend.

THERAPIST: Natalie, the point is that there is only *one person* in this world who can always praise herself no matter what happens. Who is that?

NATALIE: *Me.*

THERAPIST: That's right. Never, ever put yourself down. Other people will do it for you.

NATALIE: (*Giggles.*)

THERAPIST: Be your own *best friend*. Always talk to yourself in a good way. And praise your efforts. Remember, there is nothing that you can't do. Sometimes, you just *think* you can't do it. And that's not you. That's your anxiety talking.

Using Self-Control Acronyms to Facilitate Coping

Self-control acronyms have been developed to increase the saliency, power, and portability of cognitive coping strategies for anxious youth. Two widely recognized acronyms include the FEAR plan, from the Coping Cat Workbook (see Kendall, 1990), and the STOP symbol (Silverman, 1989; Silverman & Kurtines, 1996a).

FEAR plan
F: Feeling frightened (physical sensations such as stomachaches, headaches, shakiness)
E: Expecting bad things to happen (worries, negative self-statements, cognitive distortions)
A: Actions and attitudes (coping self-talk, problem solving)
R: Results and reward (self-evaluation, self-reward)

STOP symbol
S: Scared?
T: Thoughts? (fearful in nature)
O: Other thoughts? (coping in nature)
P: Praise (self-evaluation, self-reward)

Both self-control acronyms have been shown to be effective for anxious youth (FEAR plan: see Albano & Kendall, 2002; STOP symbol: see Eisen & Kearney, 1995; Eisen & Silverman, 1993, 1998). We prefer the STOP symbol because it cues youngsters to *stop* thinking in unhealthy ways. Given our emphasis on anxiety and temperamental features, we have expanded the STOP symbol in several ways.

Expanding the STOP Symbol

First, the *S* now stands for any of the following that needs to be addressed:

   S: Scared? (anxious, worried, nervous, frightened)
   S: Steamed? (angry, mad, frustrated)
   S: Sad? (lonely, unhappy, tearful)

The *T* continues to represent *thoughts* but in a broader context (i.e., fearful, angry, or sad). To keep things simple, we refer to the *T* as the *bad* thoughts. Once youngsters identify the relevant emotion and their unhealthy thoughts, we then encourage them to say, "I have to STOP thinking *that way*."

The *O* continues to represent *other thoughts*. To keep things simple, we refer to the *O* as the *good* (coping) thoughts. This is the hard part. Teaching youngsters to think in healthy ways does not come easily. Through modeling, role playing, and the constructive evaluation of exposures, healthy thinking eventually becomes part of the youngster's coping repertoire.

The *P* continues to represent *praise*. We encourage youngsters to get into the habit of saying, "I am proud of myself." Self-praise is based on a willingness to try and to experience partial successes. Depending on the youngster, the *P* could also mean, "I don't have to be *perfect*" (e.g., a youngster with comorbid obsessive–compulsive disorder). Finally, as youngsters' reality-test their faulty beliefs, the *P* could also represent (lack of) *proof* to support separation-related fears or worries.

Clinical Tip

For older children and adolescents, we recommend that perceived failures should be framed in terms of effort, disappointment, and future partial successes. For example, due to overwhelming fear, a youngster may not even attempt a separation-related exposure. In this case, first emphasize *effort*: that is, the youngster was *thinking about* doing the exposure. Second, emphasize that it's okay to be disappointed. In fact, disappointment is an appropriate response and much better than overwhelming anger and/or sadness. Third, discuss future partial successes to avoid a focus on failure and to inspire the youngster to make greater coping efforts. Coach the youngster to evaluate exposures along these lines: "I'm disappointed that I didn't take the school bus, but I did walk to the bus stop. I'm proud of myself. If I keep practicing, I'm going to do it."

Making the STOP Symbol Salient

To enhance the saliency and portability of the STOP symbol, we recommend using STOP sign photographic stickers (if available at your local stationery store) or having youngsters draw their own STOP symbols. These symbols, in varying sizes, can be placed in vulnerable areas that trigger separation anxiety, anger, or sadness, to facilitate a youngster's coping (see Chapters 8–10 for suggestions).

The Prescriptive Use of the STOP Symbol

The STOP symbol can also be helpful for youngsters who experience both cognitive and somatic symptoms. For example, once the youngster says, "I have to *stop thinking that way*" (following the S and T), encourage him or her to practice the breathing and progressive relaxation exercises in an unobtrusive way. Once the physical sensations are contained, the youngster is in a better position to think in constructive ways.

The STOP symbol can also be used for youngsters who experience primarily somatic symptoms, low frustration tolerance, or sadness but do not yet verbalize bad thoughts. Here, the STOP sign (without the acronym) can cue youngsters to *stop* crying and getting frustrated and to practice the developmentally appropriate relaxation sequence instead (see Chapter 4). In Dialogue 5.4, we help Natalie cope with her separation anxiety by using the STOP symbol.

Dialogue 5.4

THERAPIST: Natalie, let's go back to the birthday party and see if the STOP sign can help you cope.

NATALIE: (*Sighs.*)

THERAPIST: Why are you Scared?

NATALIE: I don't want to go to the party.

THERAPIST: What are your bad Thoughts?

NATALIE: My mom will make me get out of the car. What if she leaves me there? What if she forgets to pick me up?

THERAPIST: What should you say to yourself?

NATALIE: (*Trying to think, getting frustrated.*)

THERAPIST: (*Holds up STOP sticker.*) I have to _____ thinking that way.

NATALIE: *Stop.*

THERAPIST: Good. What is the *O*?

NATALIE: (*Pursing her lips, grimacing*)

THERAPIST: If the *T* is for the *bad* thoughts, the *O* is for the _____

NATALIE: *Good thoughts* (*looking reassured, calming down*).

THERAPIST: That's right. What were you saying to yourself when your mom told you that she would be right back?

NATALIE: I don't know (*on the verge of tears*). I would *never* see her again.

THERAPIST: And when you thought *that way*, what did you do?

NATALIE: I wouldn't let her (*mom*) go.

THERAPIST: Natalie, if you don't let your mom leave you, how will you find out that nothing bad will happen to her and that *she will* pick you up?

NATALIE: (*Shrugs her shoulders.*)

THERAPIST: Just because you *think* she will forget to pick you up, does that mean it's true?

NATALIE: No . . .

THERAPIST: What could you say to yourself instead?

NATALIE: (*Shrugs her shoulders again.*)

THERAPIST: How about, my mom *always* comes back.

NATALIE: (*Smiles.*)

THERAPIST: Is this true?

NATALIE: (*Nods her head.*)

THERAPIST: If you let your mom leave even for 1 minute, what should you say to yourself?

NATALIE: I'm *Proud* of myself.

THERAPIST: Good. Now I know *right now* that you don't believe that your mom will always come back. Let's be a detective and get some *Proof* so that you will have many *good* thoughts to help you cope.

Complementing Self-Control with Cognitive Therapy

Don't worry. Everything will be okay. Simple reassurances, at best, may temporarily "take away" a youngster's anxiety. But such reassurances do not acknowledge the youngster's concerns, nor do they facilitate coping. If anything, they encourage the separation-anxious child to become more dependent on the reassurer. Your role is to help youngsters learn to *reassure themselves.* This can be accomplished by asking youngsters probing questions and by performing tests of evidence. We illustrate with common cognitive therapy and problem-solving exercises.

"What Is the Evidence?" Technique

The "What Is the Evidence?" technique (Beck, Rush, Shaw, & Emery, 1979) helps youngsters identify fearful, negative thoughts and to develop coping cognitions. Coping thoughts inspire action. Examples include "What can I do now?" (Kendall & Chansky, 1991, p. 174). You can inspire action by asking youngsters to be detectives who are searching for evidence for and against their beliefs. In Dialogue 5.5, we help Natalie examine the evidence for and against her fear/belief that her mother will have a car accident.

Dialogue 5.5

THERAPIST: Natalie, what are you worried about?

NATALIE: My mom has some errands to do. She wants me to stay with my grandma. What if she gets into a car accident?

THERAPIST: *What is the evidence for this?*

NATALIE: She was late last time [picking me up].

THERAPIST: Did she get into a car accident?

NATALIE: No . . . but she could have. Mom's a nervous driver.

THERAPIST: *What is the evidence against your mom getting into a car accident?*

NATALIE: She has been driving for a long time.

THERAPIST: Yes . . .

NATALIE: *No accidents?*

THERAPIST: That's right. How likely is it that your mom will *actually* get into a car accident? Can you give me a percentage?

NATALIE: *Fifty percent?*

THERAPIST: That means, every other time your mom drives she will get into an accident. Is that the case?

NATALIE: (*Shakes her head.*)

THERAPIST: What does the *evidence* suggest?

NATALIE: *Ten percent?*

THERAPIST: Sounds better. But that means that every *10* times your mom gets in the car, she will have one accident. What do you think?

NATALIE: (*Holds up two fingers.*)

THERAPIST: Two percent. Good . . . but I think it's more like (*makes a 0 with fingers.*)

NATALIE: *Zero.*

THERAPIST: Is there any evidence that your mom will get into a car accident today?

NATALIE: No . . . but I'm still scared.

THERAPIST: What can you say to yourself?

NATALIE: (*Shrugs her shoulders.*)

THERAPIST: You said your mom is a nervous driver. Do you mean careful and cautious?

NATALIE: (*Nods her head.*) She drives *so slowly*. It takes us forever to go places.

THERAPIST: That's frustrating. But a careful driver is less likely to . . .

NATALIE: (*Interrupts.*) *Get into a car accident.*

THERAPIST: (*Smiles.*) So what can you say to yourself when you're worried about your mom having a car accident?

NATALIE: (*Makes a 0 with her fingers.*)

THERAPIST: No evidence and . . .

NATALIE: *She's a slowpoke.*

"What If?" Technique

What's the worst thing that could happen? Do you ever think this way? Could it have been the last time you thought about flying? Did you get on the plane? If so, you were able to separate your irrational fears from your rational mind. No such advantage exists for the anxious child. The irrational outcomes are his or her only reality (Barlow, 1995). Given the separation-anxious child's tendency to catastrophize and focus on failure, it's not surprising that he or she shows resistance to separation-related exposures. With your guidance, separation-anxious youngsters can learn to realize that even the most dreaded outcomes will not result in unrelenting doom.

Comment

The "What If?" technique (Beck et al., 1979) is easy to implement for largely innocuous separation-anxious fears (e.g., being alone when family members are present in the house). The worst thing that could happen might be feeling uncomfortable—and, remember, you *want* youngsters to *experience* anxiety. Of course, when more harrowing fears predominate (e.g., abandonment, abduction, death), anxious apprehension may prove too overwhelming. For this reason, you can substitute "What's the worst thing that could happen?" with "What's the most likely thing that could happen?" or "What's the best thing that could happen?" (Beck, 1995).

The "What Is the evidence?" technique helped Natalie realize that there was virtually no basis for her fear. In Dialogue 5.6, we help refocus her worries on more realistic, less dreaded outcomes. We continue with our car accident example.

Dialogue 5.6

THERAPIST: *What's the most likely thing that could happen?*

NATALIE: Mom will get into a car accident.

THERAPIST: Are you sure? How much evidence was there for that?

NATALIE: (*Tries not to smile, looks down, then makes a 0 with her fingers.*)

THERAPIST: What usually happens when mom leaves you with someone else?

NATALIE: *She picks me up late.*

THERAPIST: How often does she pick you up late? Give me a percentage?

NATALIE: *Ninety percent.*

THERAPIST: That means every 10 times your mom picks you up, she is late 9 times. Is that the case?

NATALIE: (*Shakes her head.*)

THERAPIST: Natalie, do you remember the *last* time your mom picked you up late?

NATALIE: At school . . .

THERAPIST: How long ago was that?

NATALIE: (*Purses lips, looks down.*)

THERAPIST: Was it last week?

NATALIE: (*Shakes her head.*)

THERAPIST: Last month?

NATALIE: *I don't remember.*

THERAPIST: Can you think of *any other* times when your mom picked you up late?

NATALIE: (*Shakes her head.*)

THERAPIST: So, *what's the most likely thing that could happen* when your mom picks you up?

NATALIE: (*Speaks in a soft voice.*) She will be on time.

THERAPIST: I didn't hear you.

NATALIE: *SHE WILL BE ON TIME.*

THERAPIST: That's right. Do you remember how long you had to wait at school when she was late?

NATALIE: I wasn't the *first* to be picked up.

THERAPIST: Are you *usually* the first to be picked up?

NATALIE: *Yes* . . . Mom promises to be early [at school].

THERAPIST: *What's the best thing that could happen?*

NATALIE: My mom will be early.

THERAPIST: *What's the worst thing that could happen?*

NATALIE: I won't be the first to be picked up.

THERAPIST: Is that okay?

NATALIE: I guess so . . .

THERAPIST: Good.

Comment

You may have noticed that we didn't start the Socratic dialogue with "What's the worst thing that could happen?" If we had, Natalie's anxious apprehension may have spiraled as she responded with answers such as "Mom would get hurt or killed." However, once her worries were redirected to emphasize *unlikely lateness*, she was ready to respond to the more loaded question. Also, as long as Natalie's mother continues to promise to pick her daughter up on time (safety signal) and follows through (parental accommodation), Natalie's anxiety will be kept to a minimum. How will Natalie cope if her mother is late? Parental accommodation and eliminating safety signals are discussed in subsequent chapters (Chapters 6, 9, and 10). For now, let's focus on teaching youngsters how to problem solve.

Becoming a Problem Solver

Thinking about potential catastrophic outcomes in constructive ways certainly helps to diminish separation anxiety. However, youngsters still need to *take action* to avoid feeling powerless. Helping youngsters learn to identify problematic areas and generate alternative solutions empowers them to take action (Barkley, Edwards, & Robin, 1999; D'Zurilla, 1986; Eisen & Kearney, 1995; Zarb, 1992). In Dialogue 5.7, we *examine the alternatives* (see Beck et al., 1979) with Natalie and help her problem-solve regarding peer-related issues.

Dialogue 5.7

Problem identification

THERAPIST: Natalie, do you have friends?

NATALIE: Not really . . .

THERAPIST: Do you have a best friend?

NATALIE: (*Looks down, nods her head.*) *Not anymore.*

THERAPIST: If you could, would you like to have more friends?

NATALIE: (*Sighs, shakes her head.*)

THERAPIST: Why do you think you have trouble making friends?

Dysfunctional interpretation

NATALIE: *No one* likes me.

THERAPIST: Why do you think that?

NATALIE: *No one* calls me.

Alternative explanations

THERAPIST: What happened with your best friend?

NATALIE: (*Purses her lips, looks down.*) She invited me to her birthday party.

THERAPIST: Did you go?

NATALIE: (*Looks up, rolls her eyes.*) *It was a sleep-over.*

THERAPIST: Does your friend *know* that you get scared?

NATALIE: *Nooo* . . .

THERAPIST: What might she think?

NATALIE: (*Shrugs her shoulders.*)

THERAPIST: What would you think if your friend didn't come to your party?

NATALIE: (*Stern expression*) *She didn't want to be my friend.*

THERAPIST: Is it possible that your friend thinks that about you?

NATALIE: (*Sad expression; nods her head.*)

THERAPIST: So Natalie, is it true that no one wants to be your friend?

NATALIE: No. I'm just scared . . .

Dysfunctional actions

THERAPIST: What do you do when someone asks you to come over?

NATALIE: (*Quickly interjects.*) *Busy* . . .

THERAPIST: What do you mean?

NATALIE: *Homework.*

THERAPIST: Do you really have *that much* homework?

NATALIE: (*Shakes her head.*)

THERAPIST: What about on the weekends?

NATALIE: Stuff . . . You know, with my family.

THERAPIST: What would you think if other kids always told you that they were busy?

NATALIE: Didn't want to be my friend.

THERAPIST: That's right. Do you *want* to get your friends back?

NATALIE: (*Nods her head.*)

THERAPIST: Can you keep running away from your anxiety?

NATALIE: No.

Alternative actions

THERAPIST: So, what can you do differently?

NATALIE: (*Shrugs her shoulders.*)

THERAPIST: Could you go on the sleep-over?

NATALIE: *I can't do that.*

THERAPIST: Remember, there is nothing that you can't do. Sometimes you just think you can't do it. Will you try?

NATALIE: My mom has to stay with me.

THERAPIST: Do any of the moms stay?

NATALIE: No . . .

THERAPIST: What else could you do?

NATALIE: Take her cell phone.

THERAPIST: What would you be doing if you did that (*makes running motions*)?

NATALIE: (*Sarcastic tone*) Running away from my anxiety.

THERAPIST: (*Smiles.*) How about one phone call?

NATALIE: Am I in jail?

THERAPIST: (*Smiles again.*) And, remember, you can only call to tell her about the sleep-over, *not to beg her to come pick you up.*

NATALIE: (*Grumbles.*)

THERAPIST: What else could you do?

NATALIE: I don't know?

THERAPIST: What have we been working on?

NATALIE: Practice the STOP?

THERAPIST: That's right. You could even take a STOP sticker with you. Keep the sticker in your pocket. You may never have to take it out. Just knowing you have the sticker to help you cope could be enough. And, remember, we're going to do this at your own pace. We have time to get you ready for a sleep-over, but you have to start doing things with your friends again.

NATALIE: What about my mom?

THERAPIST: For now, she can be around. But the idea is to have her spend less and less time with you. I want *you to learn* to take away your anxiety, not by avoiding play dates or parties or having your mom stay with you, but by practicing the exercises. Are you ready to get started?

NATALIE: I'll try.

THERAPIST: Great.

Comment

The cognitive therapy and problem-solving exercises should now become part of the STOP acronym. The *O* (other thoughts) now represents more realistic outcomes based on the evidence. As part of the *O,* ask youngsters, "Any evidence? What's the most likely thing that could happen?"

In addition, the *O*, also is the time for youngsters to think of alternative solutions to help them cope: "What can you do?" By combining the exercises, the STOP symbol becomes a concrete and compact coping tool, packed with power. The result is an enhanced perception of control in separation-anxiety-related scenarios.

Cognitive Rehearsal

Consider spending two or three sessions teaching and reviewing the cognitive therapy and problem-solving exercises. During these sessions, select increasingly anxiety-provoking scenarios from the separation-anxiety hierarchy (see Chapter 8). As a first step, help youngsters visualize all the details and obstacles they will likely confront during an in vivo exposure (see Chapters 9 and 10). With your guidance, youngsters can imagine successfully applying the cognitive exercises in specific separation-anxiety-related scenarios. Visualization is more than half the battle. *If you think you can cope, you can.* This view is a far cry from catastrophizing and focusing on failure.

Homework

Once treatment begins and it becomes clear that a youngster is prone to worry and negative self-statements, replace the "What's Happening to Me?" DD with our "Coping with My Worries" record (see Handout 5 in Appendix II). This measure helps youngsters record their worries, consider their impact, and adopt self-control strategies (i.e., coping thoughts, self-reward).

PART IV

TEACHING PARENT COPING SKILLS

In Part IV we present guidelines for teaching and practicing parent coping skills in a step-by-step fashion. Chapters 6 (education) and 7 (contingency management) are presented as independent modules, so that you can prescriptively select specific exercises or procedures based on the dimensions of separation anxiety, developmental level, or comorbid problems. In these chapters we revisit Brian (Chapter 6) and Natalie (Chapter 7) and their parents. We also introduce our fourth case example, a 12-year-old Hispanic boy, Michael, and his parents, Mr. and Mrs. M.

Michael is afraid to sleep in his own bed at night. His fear of being alone was precipitated by a neighborhood robbery that occurred 3 weeks prior to the assessment. Since the incident, Michael has demanded to sleep in his parents' bed. Any protests on his parents' part are met with explosive outbursts. Although Mr. and Mrs. M. both felt treatment was warranted, Mr. M.'s involvement did not extend beyond the parent consultation.

Data Check

Data from both the SAAS-C and SAAS-P suggested that Michael's FBA was due to his generalized anxiety (WCE) and the frequency of actual calamitous events (FCE). Data from the ADIS-C and -P, RCMAS, and MASC supported DSM-IV diagnoses of GAD and SAD. Michael's chief safety signal was his mother's presence at night. The prescriptive treatment of choice is cognitive-based procedures.

CHAPTER 6

Parent Coping Skills I

Understanding My Child's Separation Anxiety

> Brian can watch TV in his room [by himself], but when I ask him
> to brush his teeth or take a bath [alone] he refuses and throws a tantrum.
> He's manipulative.
>
> —MR. P.

THE ART OF PARENTING

Let's face it: We're living in an uncertain world. Most parents are concerned about the enormity and magnitude of the stressors that confront their children. At times, parents of separation-anxious youth may wonder what they've done wrong. We want to make one point very clear. *It's no one's fault.* As parents ourselves, we recognize that parenting is an art and not a science, and can be a formidable challenge.

By now you recognize that separation anxiety and related problems are the result of many influences. Your goal is to help parents understand the nature of their youngster's separation anxiety. By doing so, a youngster's struggles become less personal and threatening. In this chapter we show you how to help parents empower their youngsters to negotiate separation anxiety—but first we must address the issue of spousal blame, which is neither healthy nor constructive, and can certainly sabotage the treatment outcome.

No Need for Blame

A youngster's persistent separation anxiety can leave a parent feeling guilty, frustrated, and helpless. Anger and frustration are often the result of ineffective limit setting and/or friction between spouses. It's not uncommon for the "breadwinner" to implicitly blame the "homemaker" for a youngster's separation anxiety. After all, in his or her view, it is only with the spouse that the child struggles. In reality, however, the separation anxiety may be a function of the nonprimary caregiver's absence or lack of involvement.

For this reason, be sure to take a supportive stance early in the treatment process. Your initial goals are to validate parental anxieties, concerns, and frustrations, and to address any blame between partners. In Dialogue 6.1 we help Brian's parents support each other.

Dialogue 6.1.

MRS. P.: I know you think it's all my fault (*Looking at husband.*)

MR. P.: (*Sighs.*) I don't think there is a problem.

MRS. P.: That's because you let Brian fall asleep with you downstairs [watching television].

THERAPIST: There is no need for blame. It sounds like Brian is giving you (*looking at both parents*) a tough time. I'm really pleased that you're here. Most parents wouldn't consider bringing their child in for treatment until much later. It's clear that you love Brian and are sensitive to his signals. We're going to have to work together to help Brian.

MR. P.: (*Sighs, gives his wife a hesitant nod.*)

THERAPIST: You (*looking at both parents*) can have different ideas about raising your children, but when it comes to helping Brian negotiate his separation anxiety, you need to be on the same wavelength. You're a team. I look forward to working together.

Comment

The issues surrounding spousal blame, for the most part, remain the same even if only one parent participates. The noninvolved parent, either at home or from a distance (e.g., divorce), often blames his or her partner for a youngster's problems. What differs, however, is the noninvolved parent's willingness to set limits. For example, in the case of divorce, the noncustodial parent may be less likely to set limits. Weak limit setting may undermine the responsible parent's authority and potentially sabotage therapeutic success. The noncustodial parent is more likely to "give in" to a separation-anxious youngster's pleas. This capitulation may stem from guilt (e.g., over not being with the child on a regular basis) or an inability/lack of desire to set limits. As a result, the noncustodial parent may spend every waking *and sleeping* moment with his or her child.

Of course, having both parents participate is an ideal situation. But, remember, for whatever reason, one parent may still go through the motions. He or she may attend therapy sessions but demonstrate no *real* participation. If anything, the façade of involvement may hamper the treatment efforts.

Overall, if both parents participate, do your best to encourage them to work together as a team. For the single parent, empower him or her to set realistic limits in the face of juggling work, family, and a potentially uncooperative ex-spouse. In the next section, we discuss educating parents about the nature of separation anxiety in youngsters.

HELPING PARENTS UNDERSTAND SEPARATION ANXIETY

The parent education program begins by helping parents develop an understanding of the nature of separation anxiety and related problems. Your goals are to normalize a parent's concerns, address any misconceptions, and set the stage for positive treatment outcomes. Consider using any of the following sources of information (summarized) drawn from our parent-training protocol (Raleigh, Brien, & Eisen, 2001).

Some Facts about Separation Anxiety

Child and adolescent fears are extremely common. Surprisingly, many parents possess limited knowledge about the nature of fears and separation anxiety. Presenting some data based facts on the subject helps to normalize a parent's concerns. If anything, a parent may not feel so alone, learning that his or her struggles are hardly unique. As a result, you'll be in a better position to direct parental energies (rather than worries) toward treatment efforts. Familiarize yourself with the following facts (Raleigh et al., 2001):

- 90% of youngsters ages 2–14 report at least one fear.
- 40% of youngsters ages 6–12 report at least seven or more fears.
- Separation-related fears (see Chapter 2) are part of normal development.

- 40% of youngsters experience separation-related fears.
- SAD onset occurs around 6–8 years of age.

Manifestations of Separation Anxiety

Based on our conceptualization, separation anxiety can be expressed in a number of ways. A fear of physical illness and worry about calamitous events comprise the symptom dimensions. A parent may have difficulty distinguishing genuine from anxiety-based somatic complaints. Naturally, discrete physical symptoms (e.g., stomachache) in response to specific triggers (e.g., going to school) are easier to understand than more generalized responses (e.g., constant nausea). Brian and Felicia experienced primarily a fear of physical illness. Worry about calamitous events may also be difficult to detect, especially if a youngster possesses a behaviorally inhibited temperament. Natalie (introduced at the end of Chapter 4) and Michael (introduced in the Part IV introduction) primarily experienced worry about calamitous events.

The fear of being alone and the fear of abandonment capture the avoidance components of separation anxiety. For some youngsters, however, behavioral avoidance may appear limited. For example, Natalie (who feared abandonment) *could attend* most activities. Of course, her mother needed to be present or had to promise to pick her up on time. If her mom even hinted about dropping her off, a tantrum ensued.

Similarly, some youngsters may show minimal signs of overt separation anxiety. Parental accommodation is usually the culprit. As you gradually eliminate safety signals and strive to minimize parental accommodation, a youngster's separation anxiety will increase. Your role will be to educate parents about the interplay between a youngster's separation anxiety symptoms and behavioral avoidance. It is particularly important to help parents understand the impact of their own behavior during this process (to be discussed). Keep in mind the following manifestations of separation anxiety in your discussions:

- Bodily reactions
- Fearful thoughts
- Behavioral avoidance
- Reliance on safety signals

Impact of Separation Anxiety

If an individual fears flying, is that a sufficient basis to seek treatment? *It depends.* Is travel limited to an occasional vacation or is it routinely required for business? Naturally, the second scenario poses the greatest interference and would likely warrant treatment. But even infrequent events can be problematic if one responds in an intense fashion. (Think of a youngster who fears needles going for a blood test.) When gauging interference in functioning, be sure to take into account both the *frequency* and *intensity* of a youngster's reactions.

Regarding separation anxiety, interference in functioning may affect several spheres (e.g., school, family, peers) or be limited to one situation or setting. In our experience, the intensity of a youngster's reactions (rather than the frequency or pervasiveness) is usually the best indicator of the degree of distress.

For example, in comparison to Michael, Brian's separation anxiety appears to cause greater interference in functioning. Brian's fear of being alone is clearly more pervasive, whereas Michael's fear occurs only at night. But Michael, undoubtedly, will be more difficult to treat. Why is this the case?

In working with Brian (see Chapters 8 and 9), we should first address his daytime fears, then build momentum to tackle the nighttime routine. Once he has mastered his daytime difficulties, Brian will be more confident to confront his fear of sleeping alone. For Michael, however, no such advantage exists. In addition, given the traumatic flavor (i.e., neighborhood robbery) of his separation anxiety, even the most basic exposures will be highly anxiety provoking.

Being fully familiar with the variety of presentations of separation anxiety (and their impact) across childhood and adolescence will help you set realistic goals for how treatment will proceed and unfold. You will also be in the best position to select the most meaningful treatment targets to help ensure positive treatment outcomes (see Chapter 8). Be sure to address the following spheres when gauging interference in functioning:

- School
- Family
- Peers
- Extracurricular activities

The Nature of Separation Anxiety

We know that the *expression* of separation anxiety and related problems is the result of child, parent, and environmental factors interacting in a reciprocal fashion (Barlow, 2002; Ginsburg & Schlossberg, 2002; Ollendick, 1998). What's more difficult to understand, however, is the unique *underlying relationship* between biological and psychological vulnerabilities for any given youngster.

Parents will want you to be specific about the nature of their child's separation anxiety. *What is the underlying cause?* A parent may frantically search for the one event that changed the course of his or her child's life. Just like it's more acceptable to have a medical than psychological disorder, parents will find comfort in a single, easily understood event.

Sometimes a youngster's psychosocial history appears unremarkable until the precipitating event. Thus, from a parent's perspective, it actually looks like the youngster was functioning adequately. However, the precipitating event is likely to serve merely as the *trigger*. The expression of separation anxiety is ultimately the result of developing biological (e.g., temperament, anxiety sensitivity) and psychological (e.g., attachment, perception of control) vulnerabilities unfolding over time. We are suggesting that the tendencies (e.g., anxiety, worry, excessive caution, hypersensitivity to physical sensations) were *always present*. The extent to which a parent observes these tendencies is likely a function of his or her sensitivity to a child's signals.

Separation anxiety and related problems are rarely due to a single event. Try to steer parents away from limited one-dimensional points of view. Explain that separation anxiety can indeed be eliminated but that any given youngster's sensitivity to anxiety will remain, to some degree. Hence, we emphasize *managing* rather than curing a tendency toward anxious apprehension. The next step in our psychoeducational program is to help parents understand the relationship between separation anxiety and childhood behavioral problems.

HELPING PARENTS UNDERSTAND THEIR CHILD'S BEHAVIOR

In our experience, youngsters frequently differ in how they attempt to cope with separation anxiety. In response to these coping attempts, parents may view their children as manipulative, oppositional, or overly sensitive. Your goal is to help parents understand the relatively *unintentional* nature of these behaviors and to facilitate cooperative coping efforts between parents and child.

The Manipulative Child

Mr. P. believes that Brian's behavior is manipulative because *sometimes* he can be alone (e.g., watching TV). Thus, Brian *should* be able to cope with other situations if he *wanted* to. Many parents who think like Mr. P. are minimizing their youngster's separation anxiety. The only reason

Brian can stay alone is because he is distracted. During the majority of separation-related scenarios, he experiences genuine anxiety. Of course, at other times, Brian may be guilty of manipulative behavior, particularly if his parents differ in their limit-setting abilities. This difference certainly exists in Brian's case.

We believe, however, that youngsters are not *intrinsically* manipulative. You may also regularly hear parents use other choice labels, such as *lazy* or *immature*, to describe their children's behavior. There may be some truth to these characterizations, but they are not usually representative of a youngster's overall behavior. To hold this perspective of a child is unhealthy and predisposes a parent to look for confirming evidence to support his or her views. Thinking this way also absolves parents of responsibility for their role in the process.

The Oppositional Child

It's only natural for parents to become frustrated when youngsters refuse to cooperate. The parent who believes that youngsters must confront their fears is on the right track. However, forcing youngsters to cope rarely proves helpful and may lead to escalating power struggles during separation-related scenarios. In the following example, both parent and child are desperately attempting to restore control during an exposure:

Parent

Thought: Child isn't trying.
Evaluation: Child is oppositional.
Action: Forces exposure.

Child

Thought: Something bad is going to happen.
Evaluation: Parent doesn't understand the danger.
Action: Refuses to cooperate.

If a youngster possesses a high-intensity, strong-willed (spirited) temperament, he or she is likely to respond with a meltdown. The youngster's implicit message is "I feel out of control." Alternatively, behaviorally inhibited youngsters are more likely to use passive methods of resistance. For example, a child or adolescent may try to give the impression of cooperating but will unobtrusively withdraw during the exposures.

The Overly Sensitive Child

Like the oppositional child, the overly sensitive child also possesses a high-intensity temperament. The key difference, however, is that the overly sensitive child *internalizes* (rather than externalizes) his or her separation anxiety. Parents may view these behaviors (e.g., crying, pouting) as overreactions to reasonable separation-related situations and become frustrated. Hence, the threat "Stop crying or I'll give you a reason to cry" is a too common parental remark.

As you help parents understand the relationship between a youngster's separation anxiety and temperamental style, behavioral protests will be perceived as less personal and threatening. The next step, of course, is to help parents understand their *own* behavior.

HELPING PARENTS UNDERSTAND THEIR OWN BEHAVIOR

We know that parents of anxious youth are more likely to experience anxiety disorders than parents of nonanxious youth (Beidel & Turner, 1997; Fyer, Mannuzza, Chapman, Martin, & Klein, 1995; Last, Philips, & Statfield, 1987). The mechanism may be genetic, in the form of a general neurotic factor (e.g., Andrews, 1995), and/or environmental, as part of the family context (Barrett, Dadds, & Rapee, 1996; Hudson & Rapee, 2001). The most relevant family maintenance factor for parents of separation anxious youth is overprotection (Eisen et al., 1998).

It's only natural for parents to want to protect their children from situations that are beyond their developmental level or are exceedingly disturbing. However, there is a fine line between *smart parenting* and *overprotection*. Some ways parents may overprotect their youngsters include:

- Limit participation in certain activities (e.g., contact sports, sleep-overs, funerals)
- Block sources of information (e.g., newscasts)
- Conceal unpleasant circumstances (e.g., family issues, illness)

Parental overprotection is usually executed with good intentions. However, if it occurs too frequently, it may leave a child with a limited repertoire of skills and make him or her even more vulnerable to separation anxiety. The parent's message to the youngster is, "I don't think you can handle this." Of course, it's more a matter of parental anxiety. The real message is, "I don't want to worry about you—I need to know that you're safe."

Explain to parents that youngsters need to experience some anxiety, frustration, and disappointment. Only by experiencing a variety of situations does a youngster learn how to cope. Loving parents may inadvertently prevent their children from having the experiences necessary to develop competence and a sense of control. Remind parents repeatedly that *the only way to overcome anxiety is to experience anxiety*. Gently discuss the specific ways in which they are overprotective and the impact on youngsters. Help parents to make decisions based on their values and instincts, *not their anxiety*. More importantly, help parents learn to view potentially anxiety-provoking scenarios as opportunities for their youngsters to develop coping skills. In the next section, we examine the dimensions of parental overprotection more fully.

THE DIMENSIONS OF PARENTAL OVERPROTECTION

Parental overprotection is associated with higher levels of child anxiety, in general (Hudson & Rapee, 2001; Rapee, 2002), and separation anxiety, in particular (Eisen et al., 1998, 2003; Neuhoff et al., 2003). The dimensions of overprotection typically take two forms: *indulgence* and *control* (Parker, 1990; Thomasgard & Metz, 1993). We discuss both dimensions of overprotection and their relationship to childhood separation anxiety.

Indulgence

The overprotective indulgent parent–child relationship is often characterized by an anxious-insecure parental attachment to the child (Thomasgard & Metz, 1993). The indulgent parent is more likely to appease or accommodate a youngster's separation anxiety (i.e., enable avoidance behavior), particularly if a youngster has a behaviorally inhibited temperament. Alternatively, weak limit setting is likely to be the norm if a youngster possesses a high-intensity, strong-willed temperament. In both scenarios, a youngster's separation anxiety is genuine. The parent may wish to set limits (i.e., encourage exposures) but is too afraid to upset the child. As a result, the parent may experience anxiety, guilt, and anger, at times (Thomasgard & Metz, 1993).

Mrs. M. could best be characterized as an overprotective indulgent parent. She understood that Michael needed to be exposed to separation anxious events. However, her own anxiety, guilt, and need to "not upset him" stood in the way. Any hint of limit setting on her part was met with fierce resistance from Michael. In Chapters 8–10, we tackle the challenge of empowering Mrs. M. to set clear and consistent limits with her son. We also work hard to help Michael understand and accept the need for separation-related exposures.

Control

In contrast to the overprotective indulgent parent, the overprotective *controlling* parent is viewed as too vigilant and restrictive (Thomasgard & Metz, 1993). The controlling parent is more likely to attempt separation-related exposures with a youngster. However, the controlling parent may go overboard with his or her help and be viewed as too intrusive (e.g., Hudson & Rapee, 2001). Compliance is more likely if a youngster possesses a behaviorally inhibited temperament. However, the youngster may become withdrawn or respond with an avoidant style of coping (Rapee, 2002)—usually passive forms of cheating during the exposures (see Chapters 9 and 10).

Alternatively, escalating power struggles are likely to ensue if a youngster possesses a high-intensity, strong-willed temperament. The controlling parent may experience overt anger and resentment as the youngster resists his or her efforts, especially if a parent has difficulty understanding the true nature of a youngster's separation anxiety.

Given the nature of parental overprotection, it's not surprising that family environments in which youngsters are given minimal personal control are associated with childhood anxiety (Chorpita, Brown, & Barlow, 1998; Cobham, Dadds, & Spence, 1999; Ginsburg & Schlossberg, 2002; McClure et al., 2001; Rapee, 1997; Siqueland et al., 1996). In our experience, the more a parent struggles with his or her own anxiety/insecurity, the more likely the need to control other family members. Parental warmth may still be part of the picture, and if evident, is associated with lower levels of anxiety in youngsters (Dadds, Barrett, Rapee, & Ryan, 1996).

Mrs. P.'s controlling style is representative of the kind of parental dynamic you are likely to encounter. A parent with an overprotective controlling style may restrict the child from participating in age-appropriate autonomous activities (e.g., sleep-over, summer camp). In the parent's mind, the child is simply not ready for these challenges. Overprotection may come across as a parent's desire to keep his or her child safe but, in actuality, stems from a parent's own fears and anxieties surrounding issues of separation and safety.

"Don't Worry, Everything Will Be Okay"

If you were on an airplane that was experiencing turbulence and you became apprehensive, which would you find more reassuring?

- Flight attendants remain calm and go about their business.
- Flight attendants appear alarmed, drop everything they're doing, and go from person to person providing reassurance that everything is okay.

Separation-anxious youngsters may look for constant comfort and reassurance. As a result, most parents will respond with support and encouragement. The parent's message is "Don't worry, everything will be okay." Reassurance typically stems from a parent's overprotective nature (e.g., minimize child's distress) or his or her own anxiety (e.g., difficulty tolerating child's distress).

Certainly, there are occasions when anyone could use a word of reassurance. Keep in mind, however, that parental reassurance is often a quick and easy attempt to *take away* a youngster's separation anxiety. No real coping on the youngster's part is occurring. Several problems may emerge for the separation-anxious youngster if the reassurance becomes too frequent or excessive:

- Develops overdependency.
- Opportunities for developing independent problem solving are severely restricted.
- Separation anxiety is reinforced.

Separation anxiety is *reinforced*? That's right. The extraparental attention conveys the message to the youngster that his or her separation-related fears are justified. Let's return to the example of the flight attendants. If the flight attendants remain calm, you may worry that they're concealing a potential catastrophe. In the second scenario, you may appreciate the flight attendant's reassurance because it validates (but reinforces) your anxiety. However, to observe the flight attendants in a state of panic is anything but reassuring. This brings us to another way parents may encourage separation anxiety.

"Do What I Say, Not What I Do"

Which parental behavior is more likely to influence adolescent/young adult smoking?

- Repeated lectures on the hazards of smoking
- Parental smoking

If a parent smokes, lecturing about its hazards is of minimal value. A parent may inadvertently model separation anxiety in the following ways:

- Avoidance behaviors
- Fearful reactions
- Anxious postures

Parents of anxious youth are more likely to model anxiety and reinforce avoidant solutions than parents of nonanxious youth (Barrett, Rapee, et al., 1996; Chorpita et al., 1996; Hirshfeld, Biederman, Brody, & Faraone, 1997). So, if a parent acts in a fearful way, telling a youngster not to worry is hardly reassuring. The fearful model is more salient.

An anxious parental model is not limited to the *things that parents do*. The beliefs and expectations a parent holds about his or her life experiences may also contribute to a youngster's anxiety. For example, mothers of anxious youth reported lower expectations for their children's academic, social, and future success outcomes (Eisen, Spasaro, Brien, Kearney, & Albano, 2004). In addition, mothers of anxious youth rated their youngsters as *more* likely to experience anxiety and *less* likely to cope in distressing situations (Kortlander, Kendall, & Panichelli-Mindel, 1997).

Overall, it is clear that parents may engage in behaviors that *enhance* anxiety in children and adolescents (Cobham, Dadds, & Spence, 1998; Ginsburg & Schlossberg, 2002; Rapee, 1997; Siqueland et al., 1996). In response to this reality, family-based treatment programs for anxious youth have proliferated (Barrett, Dadds, et al., 1996; Knox, Albano, & Barlow, 1996; see Mattis & Pincus, 2004; Shortt, Barrett, & Fox, 2001). In the next section, we discuss our prescriptive approach to parent training for parents with separation-anxious youth.

THE PRESCRIPTIVE BASIS
FOR PARENTING TRAINING

Recently, Eisen and colleagues (Eisen et al., 2003; Neuhoff et al., 2003; Raleigh et al., 2001) developed and examined the preliminary efficacy of a 10-week integrated parent training program specifically designed for youngsters with separation anxiety. The program emphasized psychoeducation and training parents to *actually implement* cognitive-behavioral treatment strategies (i.e., relaxation training, cognitive therapy, contingency management, exposure) with their youngsters. In contrast to previous research (Cobham et al., 1998; Dadds et al., 1996), the delivery of child-based coping skills was thus *therapist-assisted*.

In the first study (Eisen et al., 2003) participants were six families with children ages 7–10 years who met DSM-IV criteria for a principal diagnosis of SAD. Using a multiple baseline design across participants (see Hayes et al., 1999), families were assessed on child, parent, and family measures at pre- and posttreatment as well as at 6-month follow-up. Daily diaries and child and parent weekly ratings monitored treatment progress. Following the assessment, each parent(s) received the 10-week flexible protocol. No further contact with any of the youngsters occurred until posttreatment and follow-up.

In general, parent training produced marked changes in parenting competence, levels of stress and anxiety, and perceptions of child symptom severity. These changes translated to major reductions in children's somatic complaints and SAD symptoms. In fact, five of six children no longer met DSM-IV criteria for SAD.

In our second study (Neuhoff et al., 2003) we examined the prescriptive utility of child cognitive-behavioral therapy versus parent training for SAD. Participants were six families with children ages 8–12 years who met DSM-IV criteria for SAD. Assessment data determined the appropriate (prescriptive) response class (child or parent) based on empirically derived clinical cutoff scores. Participants were then randomly assigned either to 10-week parent training (Raleigh et al., 2001) or child cognitive-behavioral therapy protocols (Silverman, 1989). In this way, participants either received prescriptive (i.e., elevated child anxiety with child cognitive-behavioral therapy; ineffective/anxious parenting with parent training) or nonprescriptive (i.e., elevated child anxiety with parent training; ineffective/anxious parenting with child cognitive-behavioral therapy) treatments.

In general, the results revealed that all participants improved on child, parent, and family measures at posttreatment. However, only prescriptive treatments produced substantial enough changes for participants to achieve high end-state functioning (e.g., absence of SAD diagnosis.

SELECTING PRESCRIPTIVE TREATMENTS

Naturally, your clinical judgment is the best resource for determining the ideal treatment arrangement for a given family. At the same time, however, we encourage you to give treatment selection an empirical flavor by considering the use of any of the following measures. In this section, we discuss general issues and prescriptive parent measures.

We're looking for a particular kind of parent who is likely to benefit from parent training. First, let's look at the degree of parental anxiety and overprotection; one or both parents are likely to struggle with anxiety and be overprotective. But it's a matter of degree: Moderate levels of anxiety and/or overprotection are ideal for parent training because the parent is still capable of *following through* with the program and can learn to manage his or her anxiety and degree of child involvement. Pathological levels of these variables, however, may preclude any effective form of intervention. A parent's individual therapy may be needed as a first step.

Parental Anxiety and Depression

The Beck Anxiety Inventory (BAI; Beck, 1993) and Beck Depression Inventory–II (BDI-II; Beck et al., 1996) contain 21 items, possess strong psychometric properties, and measure anxiety/panic and depression, respectively. Sample items from the BAI include "unable to relax" and "fear of losing control"; sample items from the BDI-II include "I feel sad" and "I cry more than I used to."

Parental Overprotection

The Parent Protection Scale (PPS; Thomasgard, Metz, Edelbrock, & Shonkoff, 1995) contains 25 items, has strong psychometric properties, and measures four subscales of parental protective behaviors: supervision, separation problems, dependence, and control. Sample items include "I comfort my child immediately when he/she cries" and "I keep a close watch on my child."

Comment

Based on our prescriptive model, it is also important to consider levels of parenting stress and competence. Presumably, most parents that participate in our programs are experiencing moderate to high levels of stress associated, in part, with the demands of coping with a youngster's separation anxiety (e.g., lack of sleep). In our experience, most parents may function adequately despite high levels of stress and can follow through with the program. Parents experiencing moderate to high levels of stress usually benefit from parent training.

Parenting competence is another factor to consider. A parent's confidence in his or her ability to help a youngster will play an important role in treatment. Once again, we're looking for a middle ground. Minimal confidence and low self-esteem regarding one's parenting abilities are likely to impede treatment progress. If a parent displays these qualities, consider working with the youngster as a first step. Provide as much parenting as possible as long as it remains therapeutic; too much hand holding and indecisiveness will thwart the effectiveness of the overall program. Again, if necessary, consider encouraging a parent to seek his or her own counseling as well.

Parenting Stress

The Parenting Stress Index (PSI; Abidin, 1995) contains 120 items, strong psychometric properties, and both parent and child domains. The parent domain consists of seven subscales measuring depression, attachment, role restriction, sense of competence, social isolation, relationship with spouse, and parental health. The child domain consists of six subscales that measure adaptability, acceptability, demandingness, mood, distractibility, and reinforcement of parent. Given that the completion of the PSI is time consuming and generally recommended for research purposes, consider using the short form (i.e., 36 items).

Parenting Competence

The Parenting Sense of Competence Scale (PSOC; Johnston & Mash, 1989) measures parenting efficacy, satisfaction, and self-esteem and possesses strong psychometric properties. Sample items include "Being a parent is manageable and any problems can be solved" and "Even though being a parent would be rewarding, I am frustrated now while my child is at his/her age."

Data Check

How do Brian's and Michael's parents compare on these parenting measures? Mrs. P. reported moderate levels of anxiety (BAI) and depression (BDI-II) and clinical levels of parenting stress (PSI). She also reported adequate parenting competence (PSOC). She perceived herself as an effective parent but was frustrated with Brian and Mr. P.'s lack of cooperation. Mr. P. reported minimal anxiety (BAI) and depression (BDI-II), moderate stress (PSI), and high levels of parenting competence (PSOC). He perceived his spouse as largely responsible for Brian's fearful and disruptive behaviors.

In this case, the data suggesting prescriptive parent training is mixed. However, parent training would complement Brian's prescriptive relaxation/exposure regimen, given:

- Family/marital conflict
- Mrs. P.'s controlling/overprotective nature
- Mr. P.'s lack of understanding regarding his son's separation anxiety

Michael's mother, Mrs. M., reported clinical levels of anxiety (BAI), depression (BDI-II), and parenting stress (PSI), as well as marked deficits in parenting competence (PSOC). The data clearly suggest a need for parent training procedures. Given the nature of Mrs. M.'s deficits, however, she may have difficulty following through with the program (see Chapter 9).

WHAT'S NEXT?

In Chapter 7 we present step-by-step guidelines for helping parents implement contingency management procedures with separation-anxious youth. We also introduce our fifth case example, a 3-year-old Caucasian girl, Montana, and her mother, Mrs. W. Montana lives with her parents and two older brothers (ages 5 and 8). Upon awakening, she cries hysterically and then immediately vomits. Her mild reflux condition is a contributing factor. She is terrified of sleeping alone.

Data from the BAI and BDI-II suggested that Mrs. W. was experiencing moderate levels of anxiety and unremarkable levels of depression. She reported above-average competence in her parenting abilities (PSOC) but high levels of stress (PSI). She reported being overwhelmed by the responsibilities of raising three children, especially in light of disrupted sleep at night and a largely uninvolved spouse. Data from the SAAS-P suggested that Montana's FBA was limited to the nighttime and maintained by FPI. Montana's chief safety signal was her mother's presence at night. Based on the data and Montana's young age, the prescriptive treatment of choice is individualized parent training.

CHAPTER 7

Parent Coping Skills II

Managing My Child's Separation Anxiety

> Reward Michael for staying in his room [at night]? He's *12 years old.*
> He *should* be over it [the robbery] by now. Sounds like bribery to me.
> —MR. M.

THE IMPORTANCE OF REWARDS

Think of the next time you plan to reward yourself. It could be a cold drink after a vigorous workout at the gym, a new outfit for losing weight, or more money in your pocket for smoking fewer cigarettes. Often the promise of a relaxing weekend with friends motivates us to persevere throughout the week. The expectation of a concrete reward can help us through difficult moments. The same is true for youngsters. Rewards can serve as a catalyst for the following:

- Enhance motivation to overcome separation anxiety
- Encourage willingness to participate in exposures
- Stimulate coping behaviors
- Generate a sense of accomplishment
- Enhance confidence and self-efficacy
- Make the future immediate

Your first challenge was to help parents understand the *true* nature of their youngster's separation anxiety and related problems (Chapter 6). This educational component also entailed helping parents understand the impact of their own anxiety—without arousing any sense of blame.

We think you'll find that most parents are relatively sensitive to their child's separation-related signals. Sometimes, however, parental expectations are developed without taking these signals into account. We need to take these signals into account. Some parents will need reminders. Some parents may continue to have difficulty accepting your conceptualization of their youngster's areas of weakness. For this group, your next assignment may prove formidable as well. Now you must convince these parents to appreciate the value of rewards in your efforts to eliminate their youngster's separation anxiety.

"Sounds Like Bribery"

Like Mr. M., some parents express concern about using rewards during the treatment process. You can expect to hear the following phrases:

"My child *should* be able to . . ."
• Sleep alone (be alone)
• Go to a friend's house, party, school

"My child *should* be able to . . ."
• Behave
• Listen
• Be responsible

Be alert for *should* statements. They usually suggest that a parent does not fully understand the nature of his or her youngster's separation anxiety and related problems. In Dialogue 7.1 (during the parent consultation), we help Mr. (and Mrs.) M. distinguish between bribery and contingent rewards.

Dialogue 7.1

THERAPIST: It sounds like Michael is very resistant to sleeping in his own room at night. Sometimes using rewards can help encourage youngsters to try to cope with separation anxiety.

MR. M.: Reward Michael for staying in his room? He's *12 years old.* He *should* be over it [the robbery] by now. Sounds like bribery to me.

THERAPIST: It's not bribery. Please let me explain with an example. Bribery (*looking at both Mr. and Mrs. M.*) is when you're in the supermarket and your child is whining and begging you to buy all kinds of junk food. You firmly tell him no. He keeps whining. You see your best friend coming around the corner. To avoid embarrassment, you give in and let Michael have whatever he wants.

MRS. M.: (*Sighs.*)

THERAPIST: *That's bribery.* You don't feel good about what you just did. I'm talking about changing the contingencies, in advance, to make it worthwhile for Michael to try to cope with his separation anxiety. The reward will make the exposure less aversive. Remember, the only way to overcome anxiety is to experience anxiety. Once Michael realizes that he *can* stay in his room, we can phase out the tangible rewards. Being able to cope is the best reward. But if Michael refuses to be exposed, it will be extremely difficult to make progress.

MR. M.: Won't Michael expect a reward for everything he is asked to do?

THERAPIST: It's possible that he may get greedy. But that is why we will carefully select the rewards and make them contingent on more challenging exposures. The idea is not to spend a great deal of money. In fact, many of the rewards should be his favorite activities or special time with either one of you rather than just tangibles.

MR. M.: I don't know . . .

THERAPIST: I'd like to help you recognize what's hard for Michael because of his anxiety rather than just expect him to be able to do certain things. It's not personal; he's not trying to defy you. He's doing everything in his power to avoid feeling uncomfortable. We cannot force him to become fearless. But we can motivate him to try and overcome his anxiety.

MRS. M.: I'm willing to try anything (*giving husband a hopeful look*).

MR. M.: (*Sighs, then nods.*)

The Case for Separation Anxiety

Do you have a lucky charm? A rabbit's foot, special handkerchief, favorite pen or pencil? Deep down you may know it's simply superstitious, but it still makes you feel more secure. Could you part with it? Try and ask a separation-anxious child to give up his or her security blanket. It's not going to be easy, especially if the security blanket is literally wrapped around a parent.

As a result, you can expect a great deal of resistance, especially if a parent has been accommodating (i.e., overprotecting) a youngster for a long time. The idea of exposing oneself to separation-anxiety-related scenarios is anything but appealing. Younger children may not be able to appreciate the benefits of being less fearful down the road; older children and adolescents may still be reluctant to give up their security. So we need to change the contingencies. We need to motivate separation-anxious youth to be willing to expose themselves. We need to show them that becoming less fearful and more independent is worthwhile. Let's get started.

The Right Stuff

Now it's time to help parents create a reward (i.e., positive reinforcement) hierarchy for their youngster. Consider the following list of possible rewards for children and adolescents.

Common rewards for children
- Tangible items such as food, trading cards, or playthings (e.g., stickers)
- Small toys
- Access to television and video games
- Access to computer/Internet
- Privileges, such as staying up later at night
- Social activities, such as play dates
- Board games, outings, or other activities with parents
- Attention and praise

Common rewards for adolescents
- Access to social activities with peers
- Freedom from household responsibilities
- Special activities with parents
- Access to computer/Internet
- DVD/video rentals
- CDs or cassette tapes
- Favorite meals
- Clothes
- Attention and praise

Greed Is Not Good

Some youngsters may have their own ideas when it comes to receiving rewards: They may see dollar signs or tangible items that cost a great deal of money. A reward that is expensive and grand may convey the message that the reward is all that matters. As a result, the sense of accomplishment can get lost in the process.

The purpose of the reward is to stimulate youngsters to try hard to overcome their separation anxiety. Being free from fear is the *real* reward. Rewards need not be tangible items nor expensive. In fact, encourage parents to consider using primarily social and activity rewards. The few tangible items should be reserved for completing the more anxiety-provoking exposures that occur toward the end of the program.

We find it helpful to distribute the common rewards list to parents, allowing them time to add appropriate items of their own. Together, we devise a tentative list of about 10–12 items. Be sure the list includes a healthy balance of social, activity-related, and tangible rewards.

It's Worth the Wait

Wouldn't it be great if we could get paid *before* we did our work? Youngsters are likely to embrace this idea. The only difference, however, is their lack of understanding that such an arrangement is terribly unrealistic. Some overzealous youngsters may encourage their parents to do the following:

- Purchase tangible rewards, then hold until the exposures are completed.
- Give tangible, social, or activity rewards based on the promise to participate in the exposures.

Beware: Neither arrangement is feasible. Most youngsters cannot wait for a reward that is readily available (or visible). Also, once rewarded, youngsters may have minimal incentive to participate in exposures. Forget about promises. All they feel *now* is separation anxiety. You're most likely to encounter these scenarios when working with

- an overprotective indulgent parent and a high-intensity strong-willed child
- a youngster experiencing strong comorbid generalized anxiety

In both circumstances, the youngster will have difficulty waiting to be rewarded. He or she may have low frustration tolerance and/or worry that the tangible reward will no longer be available upon completing the exposure (e.g., sold out). Use these situations to help parents set limits. Your involvement naturally adds an element of accountability. In the event that a youngster resists too vehemently, reevaluate whether or not incentives should be part of the program.

Getting Creative

It's important to remember that not every youngster will respond to, or be interested in, the typical rewards outlined above. For example, let's take a look at Montana (introduced at the end of Chapter 6). Given her young age, most of the rewards suggested would be inappropriate. In addition, she is unlikely to make the connection between staying in her bed at night and receiving a reward at a later time. Her rewards structure needs to be more concrete, immediate, and enticing.

For example, we recommended a grab bag. Mrs. W. went to a novelty store and purchased numerous trinkets for under a dollar, then wrapped each item in pretty paper. Following Montana's nighttime routine, a special package was left by her door. As long as she stayed in her room, even if she awakened in the middle of the night, she was allowed to open her package in the morning. For those difficult nights that led to possible vomiting episodes, we encouraged Mrs. W. to make use of our coping strategies in extremely concrete ways (see Chapters 8 and 9).

Considering Token Economies

Token economies are useful for separation-anxious youth who respond to concrete rewards. Typically, a youngster would acquire a predetermined number of "tokens" (e.g., gold stars, smiley faces, poker chips) for appropriate coping behaviors. When enough tokens are earned, he or she may "trade in" the tokens for a valuable social, activity, or tangible reward. We recommend that the earning of tokens should be *task oriented* rather than associated with any time intervals. For example, tokens could be earned for practicing therapeutic exercises (relaxation, STOP acronym) or for appropriate social behaviors (e.g., good attitude, enthusiasm, willingness to participate).

Tokens are useful for children who have difficulty *waiting* to be rewarded and adolescents who have their eyes on *bigger* prizes. Tokens are also helpful for reinforcing and encouraging coping behaviors in settings outside the home (see Chapter 10). For example, a youngster's first response to separation may be overwhelming fear. The presence of a token, however, may *unlock* this response and encourage a readiness to cope. Tokens are portable and can easily be carried in a purse or wallet. Tokens are helpful during both planned and spontaneous (naturally occurring) exposures (see Chapters 8–10).

Clinical Tip

Try and find a positive reinforcer that is both a token and a potent reward. For example, boys are often interested in collecting the latest trend in trading cards, and girls are likely to be fond of hair (e.g., clips or barrettes) or jewelry items from novelty/discount stores. These items, dispensed one at a time, bridge the gap until larger rewards from the hierarchy can be granted (e.g., over the weekend). For some youngsters, however, these "token reinforcers" may be sufficient.

Rewarding to a Criterion

Do you know anyone who works in sales? He or she may work for months on a sale, only to receive no commission when the deal falls through. Certainly, such an arrangement hardly seems fair. On one hand, the commission (reward) has to be contingent on a successful transaction. On an emotional level, however, the individual *should* receive something for his or her efforts. How does this principle translate when working with separation-anxious youth?

Like the salesperson situation, actual rewards are contingent upon the successful completion of exposures. *Successful* simply means getting through the exposure. Youngsters are expected to become anxious and/or frustrated. That's the idea of the assignment. However, we use tokens and healthy doses of praise to acknowledge a youngster's willingness to participate and not hide behind his or her anxiety.

For example, one of the exposure-based assignments from Brian's hierarchy (see Chapter 8) was to stay alone in his finished basement for 30 minutes. During the first attempt, he stayed for 10 minutes, started to panic, and then ran up the stairs. In what context do we evaluate such an outcome? Prior to the treatment program, Brian had never been alone in the basement for *any* length of time. Thus, his efforts clearly qualify as a partial success and are worthy of praise and/or tokens. Brian will still be rewarded to a criterion; that is, he will receive a tangible, social, or activity reinforcer only after staying alone in the basement for *30* minutes.

Once a separation-related situation is mastered, create the expectation that a reward will no longer be granted for a similar situation. The event now becomes part of the youngster's repertoire. Of course, you can encourage parents to continue offering praise and/or tokens, as needed. Another reward is then negotiated for the next item on the hierarchy. This process is similar to *shaping*, which involves successive approximations to a desired response (Martin & Pear, 1983).

Don't Forget about the Siblings

It's only natural for a youngster to experience resentment when his or her sibling receives rewards for coping with separation anxiety. For this reason, encourage parents to devise similar reward systems for siblings who are close in age. Sibling issues and reward preferences are likely to differ from family to family. The important points to emphasize, however, are *effort* and *partial successes*.

GENERAL GUIDELINES FOR USING INCENTIVES

To help ensure the successful use of incentives in your program, we recommend the following basic guidelines.

- Omit any forms of reinforcement that naturally occur too frequently (no value).
- Regularly "mix up" rewards (prevent from becoming habituated).
- Reward as soon as realistically possible once exposure is completed (not before).
- Phase out tangibles, phase in social and activity rewards over time.
- Use tokens to bridge the gap until larger rewards can be dispensed.
- Use tokens to reward effort, attitude, enthusiasm.
- Reward to a criterion.
- Reward siblings (for improvement regarding their own issues).
- Stop rewards as motivation changes from extrinsic to intrinsic (resistance lessens).

As you can imagine, rewards may not be necessary or viable in some circumstances. For example, some children and adolescents who experience debilitating (e.g., OCD) and unpredictable (e.g., panic) anxiety disorders may have a strong intrinsic desire to overcome their anxiety. In fact, due to the chronic (and uncomfortable) nature of these disorders, some youngsters may *actually ask* their parents for outside help. In some cases, rewards may not be viable if:

- Parents regularly dispense rewards without any apparent function.
- Parents do not embrace the idea of using rewards to stimulate their child's coping behaviors.

- The youngster's perception of anxiety is much stronger than the value of *any* reward.
- The youngster is too greedy and/or overzealous.

Overall, use your clinical judgment in deciding whether or not rewards should be part of the therapeutic program. In our experience, two general conditions suggest rewards may prove helpful:

- Child or adolescent demonstrates resistance to exposures.
- Parent demonstrates a lack of understanding regarding the nature of a youngster's separation anxiety.

Comment

At this point, you understand the nature and importance of using tangible, social, or activity rewards to help youngsters work hard to overcome separation anxiety. Keep in mind, however, that dispensing *actual* rewards is only part of the reinforcement process. More important are a parent's verbal and nonverbal behaviors. Therefore, our next goal is to help parents *differentially* reinforce a youngster's coping efforts by becoming more effective communicators themselves.

FACILITATING EFFECTIVE PARENTAL COMMUNICATION

Are We Clear?

It's not uncommon for parents to deliver unclear commands to their youngsters. These *beta* commands (McMahon & Forehand, 2003) are vague, disrupted by other statements, or ignored by the youngster. For example, "Clean your room" does not specify how or when the room should be cleaned. As a result, noncompliance and power struggles are likely to ensue. Beta commands may also be issued in the form of questions (e.g., "Will you get ready for bed?"), or in a critical way (e.g., "Brush your teeth, for crying out loud").

Our goal is to help parents use *alpha* commands; that is, communicating their expectations in clear, unambiguous ways. "Clean your room" now becomes "Put your toys in the closet within the next 5 minutes." Alpha commands leave minimal room for misinterpretation, thus facilitating successful compliance.

Traditionally, command training has been utilized with youngsters experiencing disruptive behavioral problems (e.g., Barkley et al., 1999). How does this approach translate when working with separation-anxious youth? Let's take a look at the following examples with Natalie and her mother.

Vague approach

MRS. C.: If you stay at the party and act your age, we'll do something special over the weekend.

Comment

Natalie has no idea what is expected of her, nor does she know what reward will be received. For example, what is meant by "act your age" or "do something special"? We need to help Mrs. C. set realistic goals for her daughter (see Chapters 8 and 10) and communicate precisely what is expected of her.

Clear approach

MRS. C.: I will stay in the waiting area if you join the party [gym area] for *10 minutes*. Your reward will be dinner at Wendy's and will include a sandwich of your choice, fries, soda, and a dessert.

Comment

Will Natalie be successful? She may not stay for 10 minutes. At least now, however, she is likely to try and stay for as long as she can. Remember, partial successes based on effort are the foundation of our program. Each exposure builds momentum.

Grin and Bear It

When a separation-anxious youngster behaves in overly fearful or inappropriate ways, his or her behavior *demands* a parent's attention, and most parents respond with *anxiety-enhancing* behaviors (e.g., reassurance, physical affection, coercion) that actually *reinforce* separation anxiety and related behaviors.

One of the key purposes of contingency management is the reorientation of reward (verbal and nonverbal) from fearful to coping behaviors. So, on the one hand, you will encourage parents to largely ignore their youngster's attention-seeking behaviors, such as:

- Need for excessive reassurance
- Somatic complaints

- Whining
- Crying
- Tantrums

We see these behaviors as causing a *tolerable* level of disruptiveness. Of course, each parent will have a different threshold for ignoring *before* intervening. Some parents will literally ignore (i.e., dismiss) their youngster's behavior. Be sure to explain to these parents that they initially need to validate their youngster's concerns and *then* ignore the behaviors. In Dialogue 7.2, we continue our example with Natalie and her mother using our *V* (validate), *R* (remind of reward/prescriptive coping exercises), *I* (ignore verbal and nonverbal behaviors) acronym.

Dialogue 7.2

NATALIE: (*Clinging to Mrs. C.*)

*V*alidate:

MRS. C.: I know you're worried about me staying in the waiting area, but you have to try to join the party. (*Gently nudges Natalie forward to gym area.*)

NATALIE: (*Crying*) I can't. Don't go . . .

*R*emind:

MRS. C.: I will stay in the waiting area if you join the party for 10 minutes. Your *reward* will be dinner at Wendy's and will include a sandwich of your choice, fries, soda, and a dessert. Use your *STOP*. (*Smiles, walks back to waiting area.*)

*I*gnore:

MRS. C.: (*Talks with other parents, reads a magazine.*)

NATALIE: (*Sighs, then pulls out STOP sticker from pocket. She walks toward party, but makes sure she can see her mom at all times*).

Comment

In this scenario, Mrs. C. communicated her objectives in a clear and calm manner. At the same time, parental anxiety-enhancing behaviors were replaced with a contingent reward and prescriptive cognitive coping exercises. In contrast, some parents may have great difficulty with the *ignoring* part. For example, Mrs. M. was extremely sensitive to Michael's distress, and she couldn't conceal her own fearful facial expressions. Thus, Michael's ambivalence regarding the exposures heightened, and his resistance increased. It is important to coach parents to adopt calm verbal and nonverbal postures so that they serve as a *coping* rather than a fearful model.

Planned ignoring initially results in increased attention-getting behaviors before they subside (extinction burst). Not only are we taking away a youngster's security (through exposures), but we are also gradually eliminating the reassurances and safety signals that help him or her cope in unavoidable situations. Be sure to create this expectation. Otherwise, some parents may get frustrated, perceive a lack of progress, and terminate prematurely.

Focus on Coping

What should parents do if attention-getting behaviors endure for long intervals? Rather than resorting to overprotective or punitive methods, we recommend *shaping* a youngster's behavior. Let's take a look at an example with Montana and her mother, when Montana awakens in the middle of the night.

> ### Dialogue 7.3
> MONTANA: (*Crying hysterically, breathing shallow.*)
> MRS. W.: (*Walks into room.*)
> MONTANA: (*Gestures for her mom to get in bed with her.*)
> MRS. W.: Do your breathing.
> MONTANA: (*Takes a deep breath, gestures again.*)
> MRS. W.: Use your words.
> MONTANA: (*Cries louder.*)
> MRS. W.: (*Looks down, avoids eye contact.*)
> MONTANA: (*Continues crying.*)
> MRS. W.: (*Continues to avoid eye contact, takes a step toward the door.*)
> MONTANA: Stay . . . (*Continues crying.*)
> MRS. W.: (*Smiles.*) I'll stay. Calm down. (*Gestures to breathe slowly.*)
> MONTANA: (*Catches her breath.*)
> MRS. W.: (*Pulls up a chair next to Montana's bed.*)

Comment

In this scenario, Mrs. W. makes her positive attention (verbal and nonverbal) contingent on Montana's coping efforts. She is *showing* Montana how to get her attention in appropriate ways. It would have been easier to reprimand, reassure, or coddle Montana to stop crying. Such tactics not only would reinforce Montana's fearful behavior but also would leave her without any means to cope on her own. In Table 7.1, we show what works and what doesn't work when shaping youngsters to cope.

You now understand how to help parents shape their youngsters coping behaviors. But the rewards process is still too informal, because verbal agreements can be problematic. We need an element of accountability to make it real. In short, we need a contract.

THE ART OF THE CONTRACT

Would you seal the purchase of a new car with a handshake? Would you rent an apartment without a lease? Even simpler matters such as financing a new digital camera or leather couch may come with a contract. The contract holds both parties accountable and helps avoid potential "loopholes." The benefits of using contingency contracts with separation-anxious youth include *documentation* of:

- Task requirements during exposures
- Reward benefits
- Behaviors expected (anxious and coping)

Let's take another look at the verbal agreement between Natalie and her mother and see how a contingent contract can increase the likelihood of a successful exposure.

TABLE 7.1. Shaping Verbal and Nonverbal Behaviors

Verbal	Nonverbal
What doesn't work	
"Are you sure you're okay?"	Wincing
"You're too young for that."	Coddling
"You could get hurt."	Sighing
What works	
"You can handle it."	Smile
"Do the best you can."	Thumbs up
"How can I make it easier?"	Calm posture

Exposure: Natalie joins the party (gym area) for 10 minutes, and Mrs. C. stays in waiting area.

Reward: Dinner at Wendy's with a sandwich, fries, soda, and a dessert.

Comment

Looks reasonable? Natalie, however, wasn't satisfied. She demanded to receive her reward immediately after the party and thought that she deserved the "Biggie" size. Thus, the verbal agreement between Natalie and her mother was still *too vague*. In addition, in the absence of a written contract, either party may conveniently forget the relevant details or be less likely to follow through in a timely manner. To avoid later misunderstandings that create confusion and resentment, let's cement the deal with a contract (see Figure 7.1).

Both parties are held accountable with the contract (see Handout 2 in Appendix II for generic contract). Natalie and her mother each understand what's specifically required of her during the exposure. As you can see, the *relevant details* are extremely important. For example, *now* Natalie knows the "Biggie" size is not part of the deal. She also understands what's minimally required of her to earn a partial success. Remember, we *want* youngsters to be successful during the initial exposures to build momentum for later, more difficult challenges.

In addition, it's important to frame the contract in positive terms. For this reason, we use *do's and do's* (rather than don'ts). We also document *expected* behaviors (anxious and coping) for both parent and child during the exposure. Helping families know what to expect during exposures serves several functions:

- Enhances tolerance of anxious behaviors (child).
- Enhances awareness of anxiety-enhancing behaviors (parent).
- Encourages family members to cope (focus on do's).
- Creates a context in which exposures can be evaluated constructively.
- Facilitates realistic expectations.
- Lessens disappointment and frustration.
- Minimizes uncertainty.
- Sets the stage for family-oriented problem solving.

Prepare to Negotiate

To help ensure that the negotiation process proceeds smoothly, introduce the contract to children and their parents separately. Discuss pos-

Date: _____

Exposure-based assignment:
Natalie joins the party in the gym area for 10 minutes.
_____

_____

Specific conditions:
Mrs. C. stays in the waiting area.
_____

_____

Relevant details:
(child or adolescent)

DO: (GOAL)
Natalie stays in the gym area. She participates with the group.
_____

WHAT TO EXPECT (CHILD):
Natalie may get nervous.
_____

DO: (HOW TO COPE)
Natalie practices her STOP. She keeps a sticker in her pocket.
_____

Relevant details:
(parent)

DO: (GOAL)
Mrs. C. stays in the waiting area. She speaks with other parents
(acts natural).
WHAT TO EXPECT (PARENT):
Mrs. C. may lose patience.
_____

DO: (HOW TO HELP CHILD COPE)
Mrs. C. refrains from eye contact and/or gesturing with Natalie
until assignment is concluded.

REWARD
Success: Mrs. C. takes Natalie to Wendy's on Friday night. Natalie receives a
sandwich of her choice, medium fries and soda, and a dessert.
Partial success: Natalie receives one token/praise if she practices her STOP and/or
stays in the gym area for at least 1 minute.

Relevant signatures:

_____
(Child or Adolescent)

_____
(Parent or Guardian)

_____
(Therapist)

FIGURE 7.1. Sample Contingency Contract

sible exposure-based assignments and the rewards to be earned. Additional time may be needed to help youngsters anticipate both the demands of the assignment and the likelihood of earning rewards. Any reservations on the youngster's part may lead to modifications in the contract. Exposure-based homework assignment should be challenging but within reach, especially early in the treatment process.

Both parties should then review the final contract and voice any potential concerns. Everyone is expected to sign the contract; each is given a copy. Contracts should be displayed in visible area of the youngster's house (e.g., refrigerator). In subsequent sessions, review the outcome of the contract. Make sure everyone is on the same wavelength. Separate contracts should be paired with each exposure-based assignment (hierarchy).

Be sure to set the precedent that you will determine the manner in which rewards are dispensed if ambiguous outcomes emerge. Typically, youngsters are too lenient, so we have to help them become more accountable. Alternatively, parents may be too strict, so we need to encourage their appreciation of partial successes. Use your judgment in these scenarios and do your best to maintain the momentum of a youngster's efforts. We recommend using contingency contracts with youngsters who are at least 6 years old. Sticker charts may be more suitable for younger children.

PART V

CONFRONTING SEPARATION ANXIETY

In Chapter 8 we discuss how to structure treatment sessions with regard to skills building, hierarchy development, and treatment planning for each of our cases. More importantly, however, we help you anticipate and prepare for the therapeutic nuances that may occur as treatment unfolds.

In Chapters 9 (on fear of being alone [FBA]) and 10 (on fear of being abandoned [FAb]) we provide an intricate narrative of the process of behavioral exposure for each of our cases. We discuss the application of prescriptive child and/or parent coping skills in a step-by-step fashion. Emphasis is placed on maintaining perception of control, modifying safety signals, and overcoming resistance.

CHAPTER 8

Structuring the Treatment Sessions

Skills Building, Hierarchy Development, and Treatment Planning

SKILLS-BUILDING PHASE

The first part of the treatment program (following rapport building) should emphasize the development of prescriptive coping skills. In the next section, we provide general guidelines and tips for structuring sessions that include relaxation and cognitive procedures. Of course, elements of both can be applied, as needed, on a prescriptive basis.

Relaxation-Based Child Sessions

Consider spending one session with the youngster demonstrating the relaxation-based exercises (see Chapter 4). Pay attention to the youngster's

- Intensity
- Interest
- Attention span

Feel free to make any adjustments needed (e.g., length of script, duration of tensing and relaxation intervals) and decide whether you will record the tape (1) live in session, (2) live with concurrent therapist demonstration, or (3) outside the session.

The second session can be devoted to recording the tape live with concurrent therapist demonstration. In the event that you record the tape out of session, use this session to play, demonstrate, and practice the tape's exercises with the youngster. Finally, a third session can be used to teach and practice relaxation as a coping tool as well as to set the stage for forthcoming exposure-based homework assignments.

Clinical Tip

In our experience, most youngsters will listen to their relaxation tape. What differs is the frequency of practice and the youngster's degree of initiative. As a general rule, when working with youngsters under 10 years of age, we recommend practice-based contingent rewards to build and sustain momentum. We want youngsters to look forward to practicing their relaxation exercises rather than viewing the tape as a nuisance.

Rewards at this stage may not be as necessary for older children and adolescents, however. Of course, this will depend on the youngster's developmental level and degree of intrinsic motivation. In any case, encourage youngsters to assume as much responsibility for practicing as feasible.

Concurrent Parent Sessions

In general, be sure to cover basic relaxation principles with parents, irrespective of prescriptive treatments. For example, it is important to demonstrate the specific relaxation/breathing exercises as well as to discuss the concept of relaxation as a general anxiety-management and coping tool (see Chapter 4). It is best to create the expectation in parents that their child should listen to his or her tape regularly (i.e., at least three times per week).

In addition, encourage parents to listen to and perform the relaxation/breathing exercises initially, along with their youngsters. The goal is to help parents encourage, rather than demand, that youngsters take initiative and practice as independently as possible.

Cognitive-Based Child Sessions

Consider spending one session introducing, modeling, and practicing self-control strategies for the youngster (see Chapter 5). Be sure to discuss the importance of effort and partial success. Pay attention to the youngster's

- Attention span
- Developmental level
- Abstract thinking ability

You can make any adjustments necessary to facilitate the understanding and practice of the exercises (e.g., use cartoon strips with empty thought bubbles to be filled in, storytelling, coloring, metaphors, play therapy). During the second session, cognitive therapy and problem-solving exercises are introduced, modeled, and practiced. In general, we recommend the second sequence of exercises for youngsters 10 years and older (see Chapter 5). A third session can be devoted to practicing cognitive-based exercises as a coping tool as well as setting the stage for forthcoming exposure-based homework assignments.

Clinical Tip

In our experience, some youngsters may forget to practice the STOP acronym as a coping tool in separation-related situations. For this reason, it is best to encourage youngsters to practice *out loud* (if in an appropriate place). As with the relaxation tape, we recommend the use of practice-contingent rewards to build and sustain momentum. It is helpful to let a youngster know that you will be encouraging his or her parents to prompt the use of the exercises. Parental prompting is often viewed as intrusive and will likely increase noncompliance. As a result, it's important to clarify that prompting is not intended to annoy but to facilitate the child's ability to cope. In addition, assure the youngster that as his or her practice becomes more independent, parental prompting will decrease steadily. We also recommend that youngsters place STOP stickers or homemade acronyms in strategic areas to trigger more regular practice.

Concurrent Parent Sessions

During the parent sessions generally we find it helpful to discuss and demonstrate the specific cognitive-based exercises (e.g., STOP acronym), with an emphasis on the importance of *effort* and *partial successes*. In addition, it is important to create the expectation that youngsters, at least initially, will need to be prompted to use the exercises. Our experience suggests that parents may either be too forceful or overdo the prompting in some way. Be sure to help parents recognize the value of using a neutral tone of voice (i.e., unemotional) as well as the best times to prompt their youngsters.

FEAR OF BEING ALONE DURING THE DAY AND AT NIGHT

Hierarchy Development

Brian's Daytime Fears

Let's take a look at some common hierarchy items that are relevant for Brian and the majority of youngsters that fear being alone during the day (Figure 8.1).

Modifying the Safety Signals

You may have noticed that we omitted specific fear ratings. This is because the *context* of the exposure and the strength of the safety signal(s) will determine both the degree of anxiety and a youngster's willingness to be exposed. For example, exposures may be more or less anxiety provoking by varying

- Length of time
- Choice of safety signals
- Proximity of safety signals
- Time of day

Comment

Young children may have difficulty specifying fearful situations. You can use the fear of being alone (FBA) hierarchy as a base to start your queries. In addition, rank ordering separation-related scenarios may prove problematic for youngsters. Instead, consider asking comparative

Item	
	Less Fearful
Play in bedroom alone, with door ajar (family member(s) on same floor)	
Family room, den, kitchen alone (family member(s) on same floor)	
Bathroom alone (brush teeth or use toilet); bath or shower (family member(s) on same floor)	
Upstairs/downstairs (alone on a different floor from family members)	
Basement (finished) alone	**More Fearful**

FIGURE 8.1. Fear of being alone: Brian's daytime hierarchy items.

questions, such as, "Which is more scary for you, being alone in your bedroom with your mom down the hall or being alone in the family room with your dad in his office?"

We generally recommend using some form of a *fear thermometer* (FT; March & Mulle, 1998; Silverman & Kurtines, 1996a). The FT is a concrete tool that likens rising temperatures with "hotter" fear levels. Youngsters can draw and color their own FTs, or you could provide blank illustrations (Friedberg & McClure, 2002). For older children and adolescents, rating scales may be sufficient (e.g., 0–10 or 0–100). If you're working with parents as well, it is best to create separate hierarchies and then combine them for the most representative sample of the youngster's FBA. In the next section, we discuss our four-step plan to help youngsters stay alone during the day.

Treatment Planning

Daytime Plan

STEP 1: MAKE AN EFFORT (ANY EFFORT)

At the point of intake, most separation-anxious youngsters regularly avoid being alone. To minimize resistance during exposures, be sure to create the perception of control. It is best to start with the lowest anxiety-provoking item on the hierarchy. Treatment principles include:

- *Be gentle* regarding the length of time (exposure) and the proximity of safety signals.
- *Be firm* regarding the idea of participation (avoidance is not an option). Remember, *any effort* on the youngster's part will build momentum.

Clinical Tip

Consider setting minimum and maximum goals. Sometimes youngsters will *shut down* simply thinking about difficult exposures. If you suggest both minimum goals (i.e., youngster's idea of what he or she can handle) and maximum goals (i.e., your idea of what the youngster is likely capable of accomplishing), you will enhance a youngster's perception of control and increase the likelihood of willful participation. Typically, the outcome of the initial exposure will be somewhere in the middle.

Criterion

We find it helpful to increase the time (exposure) and distance from safety signals until mastery occurs (expected for youngster at a given age). In Brian's case, it was reasonable to expect him to stay in his room alone (door ajar) for 30 minutes before moving up the hierarchy.

STEP 2: MOVE UP THE HIERARCHY

Help the youngster decide what he or she is willing to attempt next. You can then increase the time and distance for each exposure (room for negotiation), until a minimal level of mastery is achieved.

STEP 3: CHALLENGE PERCEPTION OF CONTROL

Once a representative sample of hierarchy items has been addressed and mastered, you will need to challenge a youngster's perception of control by augmenting the perceived difficulty of exposures. The upstairs/downstairs exposure represents such an example. In Brian's case, he was now expected to stay alone on a floor (i.e., no family members present anywhere on the floor).

STEP 4: ENHANCE PERCEPTION OF CONTROL

Some exposures clearly have practical value (e.g., staying in bedroom/ bathroom alone). Other exposures, however, are designed simply to enhance perception of control. Such exposures need not become part of the youngster's repertoire. For example, some youngsters may choose to avoid spending time alone in their finished basement. At the same time, parents may not require them to do so. From our perspective, mastering such exposures often greatly enhances a youngster's perception of control. The youngster may never choose to be alone in the basement again. The fact that he or she *can be alone* in the basement is all that matters. Such exposures are helpful for negotiating separation anxiety as well as for building overall confidence. Naturally, any confidence boosters will come in handy as youngsters tackle the more challenging nighttime routine.

Nighttime Plan

Once the *key* daytime fears are addressed (see Chapter 9), it's time to target the nighttime routine. As you'll see, there are many different levels of negotiation. At intake, Brian was sleeping downstairs with his father in the family room. We think you'll find that most youngsters who have this form of separation anxiety will be sleeping in rooms other than their own (parent, sibling). Sometimes, however, a parent may sleep in his or her youngster's bedroom in a trundle bed or on the floor for the entire night. In the following material we describe our four-step process to help youngsters return to their bedrooms and stay there for the entire night.

STEP 1: BACK TO THE BEDROOM

The youngster attempts to fall asleep at night in his or her bedroom; the parent sits in a chair until the youngster falls asleep. Be sure to institute the "coach's rule": *No sleeping in other rooms.* Your rule helps keep parent and child accountable.

Comment

It's important to break the cycle in which the youngster sleeps in other rooms. Furthermore, if the parent was sleeping on the floor, he or she is now sitting in a chair. You will need to create the expectation that the parent will leave once his or her child falls asleep. Once the nighttime routine is completed (i.e., reading a story, kiss or hug), physical contact should be kept to a minimum. Most youngsters are not thrilled with this scenario but will comply as long as the parent stays until they fall asleep.

Criterion

Child does not awaken immediately when the parent leaves the bedroom.

STEP 2: THE PHASE OUT

The parent gradually phases him- or herself out of the youngster's bedroom by moving the chair away from the bed until the chair is in the hallway. The youngster's door is left ajar so he or she can still see or hear the parent. The parent stays in the hallway until the youngster falls asleep.

Comment

This step may be accomplished in one or two nights, but more typically gets negotiated over a few weeks. The difficulty of this exposure has little to do with the parent's distance from the youngster. The parent is still in his or her presence and stays in the hallway until the youngster falls asleep. It's more a function of what the distance represents *psychologically*; that is, a loss of control. Once this level gets negotiated, the youngster's perception of control is strong enough to attempt the next challenge.

Criterion

Child does not awaken immediately when the parent leaves the chair in the hallway.

STEP 3: ASSUME NORMAL NIGHTTIME ROUTINE

This is the hard part; this is the reason why the family sought your help. Following a reasonable nighttime routine, you will need to create the expectation that a parent will leave the youngster's room *before* he or she falls asleep.

Comment

At this point, most youngsters will have slept through the night (i.e., did not awaken after parent left the bedroom) a number of times. In addition, most youngsters are comfortable with the parent sitting in the hallway. The difficulty of this step is that youngsters still do not realize that they can fall asleep on their own.

In the event the youngster awakens prematurely and becomes apprehensive (e.g., shrieks, yells for parent), encourage him or her to stay in the bedroom and wait for the parent to visit. Of course, the youngsters might immediately race to the parent's bedroom with the hope of remaining there for the rest of the night. Remember your rule: *No sleeping in other rooms.* The task here is to gradually cut back the frequency of child and/or parent visits during the night.

Criterion

The youngster falls asleep on his or her own and sleeps through the night. Keep in mind that the youngster may awaken and still meet the criterion, as long as he or she stays in the room and does not cause family disruption.

Comment

The youngster may have awakened but was simply too tired to do anything about it. Sleeping alone for one night sets the stage. You want to be sure that sleeping alone becomes a regular pattern and that the youngster is practicing his or her coping skills. For this reason, we recommend *one consecutive week* of sleeping alone in his or her bedroom, with no family disruption, as the ultimate criterion.

STEP 4: ENHANCE PERCEPTION OF CONTROL

The goal here is to further enhance a youngster's perception of control by gradually eliminating other relevant safety signals (e.g., nightlight, hall light, television) that give him or her a false sense of security. Attempting to address this level depends heavily on the pace of the youngster's progress and the family's willingness to continue beyond the previous level. A youngster and his or her family can *live with* the presence of these less potent safety signals. The problem, however, is that the tendency (insecurity at night) remains. As a result, there is a greater likelihood of slips and the potential for spillage (i.e., less confidence) in other areas.

FEAR OF BEING ALONE AT NIGHT

Hierarchy Development

Michael's Initial Nighttime Fears

Unlike working with Brian, we do not have the luxury of targeting less anxiety-provoking daytime fears in our work with Michael. However, we can build Michael's confidence by first addressing nighttime fears that are not specific to sleeping alone. As you can see in Figure 8.2, some hierarchy items are relevant for most youngsters who fear sleeping alone at night. Naturally, some items are specific to the nature of Michael's separation anxiety.

Comment

Unlike Brian, Michael is afraid to be alone only at night. Younger children tend to be afraid to be alone during the day *and* night. The time of day doesn't make a great deal of difference. With older children and adolescents, however, FBA during the night is more typical. In addition, nighttime fears tend to be stronger. For example, older children and adolescents are more likely to experience strong forms of fear of

Item	
	Less Fearful
Participate in after-school activities (e.g., sports) that require coming home at night	
Upstairs/downstairs exposures	
Be the first to enter the house	
Stays in house (parent remains in garage)	
	More Fearful

FIGURE 8.2. Fear of being alone: Michael's initial nighttime hierarchy items.

physical illness (FPI; e.g., nocturnal panic attacks) and/or worry about calamitous events (WCE; generalized anxiety disorder) that maintain FBA.

Treatment Planning

Initial Nighttime Plan

We can approach Michael's initial nighttime fears in a similar fashion as Brian's daytime fears; we follow the previous sequence, starting with the item lowest on the hierarchy. First we need to create the perception of control, and targeting Michael's after-school activities is a good place to start. He was willing but apprehensive about continued participation. Because his mother was overly sensitive to his anxiety, she did not force him to attend activities if he felt uncomfortable; as a result, his attendance was slipping. For this reason, we were firm regarding attendance but conveyed no (or minimal) expectations about his performance.

As we moved up the hierarchy, we expected some resistance as Michael attempted the upstairs/downstairs exposure (i.e., being alone in either location). Maintaining his perception of control was likely to mean literally running up and down the stairs as quickly as he could. For this reason, we gradually increased the time and proximity of his safety signals until a minimal criterion was reached. In Michael's case, 5 minutes was an ambitious goal. At this point, he was likely to be willing to enter his house first (i.e., technically alone). Once again, we had to break this exposure into small steps and gradually modify his safety signals until a reasonable criterion was reached. The final exposure was attempted and negotiated to a minimal criterion (i.e., 1–2 minutes) before targeting the nighttime routine.

Nighttime Plan

Once the initial nighttime fears are addressed (see Chapter 9), it's time to target the nighttime routine. The structure for approaching the different levels of Michael's FBA at night is similar to the one we used with Brian. The process of *negotiating* these levels, however, is another story.

Michael's separation anxiety has an element of reality in it: The neighborhood robbery clearly threatened his perceived sense of personal safety. As a result, Michael was convinced that *his house* was next, and *every noise* signaled an intruder's presence.

Prior to this event, Michael's anxiety consisted largely of generalized worries involving limited avoidance behaviors. Typically, most youngsters have not experienced any actual adverse outcomes (e.g., robbery, family member's illness) that could trigger FBA. Rather, their irrational worries may amplify the perceived likelihood of calamitous media-based events or family concerns. Keep in mind, however, that actual calamitous events will make the process of cognitive therapy more challenging (see Chapter 9). In the next section, we discuss how WCE makes our four-step nighttime plan more difficult to negotiate.

The Challenges of Worry about Calamitous Events

STEP 1: BACK TO THE BEDROOM

Most youngsters will comply with the requirement to sleep in their bedroom as long as a parent stays until they fall asleep; this is also true for youngsters with FPI. The bulk of the anxiety only kicks in *if* the youngster awakens in the middle of the night.

For youngsters with WCE, however, a parent's presence until he or she falls asleep is not enough. The youngster may become so preoccupied about waking up alone that he or she remains uncomfortable even when the parent is present. As a result, the youngster may demand that the parent promise to stay for the entire night. Such a strategy is not ideal, but it is still better than allowing the youngster to sleep in other rooms, and it can be considered a first step.

As the youngster feels increasingly secure that a parent will stay (i.e., the youngster experiences an enhanced perception of control), he or she will start to fall asleep at a reasonable hour. We find it helpful to encourage parents to keep a log for 1 or 2 weeks of how long it takes for the youngster to fall asleep each night.

Comment

Once the youngster starts to fall asleep at a reasonable hour (and is not waking up), present the data from the log (e.g., falls asleep within 2 hours every night) to the youngster. You can then negotiate how long a parent can stay. A good starting point is the longest time it took the youngster to fall asleep during the last week. Of course, the youngster will become more anxious when he or she knows a parent will be leaving at night. It is helpful to create the expectation that it will take longer for the youngster to fall asleep the first few nights. Be sure to encourage parents to be flexible and not rigidly adhere to the new criterion.

Rule of thumb: Expect the youngster initially (i.e., first few nights) to require *twice* the amount of time (from criterion) to fall asleep.

Criterion

The youngster does not awaken immediately when the parent leaves his or her bedroom.

Comment

Being realistic, knowing that youngsters with WCE are likely to be hypervigilant (and consequently, less likely to fall asleep and more easily awakened), we set an attainable goal: On the first night a parent leaves the bedroom, the child does not awaken immediately. Most youngsters experience a heightened sense of control once this criterion is reached, which sets the stage for approaching the next level. When resistance is strong, encourage parents to let the youngster go to bed later (over the weekend) so that fatigue ultimately kicks in and facilitates the likelihood of success.

STEP 2: THE PHASE OUT

Naturally, you can expect some resistance here, the extent of which will be determined by the youngster's temperamental intensity and maintenance factor (FPI and/or WCE) and parenting style (see Chapter 9). Initially, the parent stays in the hallway until the youngster falls asleep. Disregard the criterion from the previous level. This task is far more challenging. The youngster is now alone and further away from his or her parent. To enhance the youngster's perception of control, the parent stays until he or she falls asleep. The implication, of course, is that a parent will stay as long as needed. Once again, encourage the parent to keep a log so that a new criterion may be established. Be flexible until the next target is reached.

Rule of thumb: Expect the youngster to require *half* as many nights (from Step 1) to fall asleep.

Criterion

The youngster does not awaken immediately when the parent leaves the chair in the hallway.

Comment

Once this criterion is accomplished, most youngsters with WCE are ready to approach the next level. Of course, when resistance is strong, this criterion may be achieved only after prolonged periods of time and/or considerable sleep deprivation. In addition, the parent's distance from the youngster's room may need to be negotiated.

STEP 3: ASSUME NORMAL NIGHTTIME ROUTINE

This level is particularly challenging for older children and adolescents who have strong forms of FPI (panic) or WCE. Youngsters with WCE are less likely to *allow* a parent to leave before he or she falls asleep; they are more likely to become hysterical and keep the entire family up for extended periods. If this is the case, you may need to substitute one safety signal (e.g., parent) with a less potent, but meaningful, one (e.g., television, radio). Your goal is for the youngster to *willingly* allow a parent to leave. In time, you can cut back (or eliminate, if necessary) the duration of the safety signal.

Youngsters with FPI are more likely to keep calling out to a parent (e.g., "I love you," "Goodnight") and expecting a reassuring response. In addition, they may repeatedly demand to go to the bathroom. Naturally, the idea is to gradually cut back parental responses to these attention-getting behaviors.

In the event that a youngster refuses to fall asleep or awakens prematurely, encourage him or her to *stay in the room* and wait for a parent to visit. Of course, some youngsters will immediately race to a parent's bedroom. In this case it is best to strongly encourage a parent to bring his or her youngster back to the bedroom. Gradually, the parent can cut back the frequency and duration of these visits. Also, do your best to encourage the youngster to stay in his or her room for longer periods of time *before* he or she visits a parent. Prescriptive coping exercises and/or rewards can be applied as stricter goals are adopted (see Chapter 9).

Criterion

The youngster falls asleep on his or her own and sleeps through the night. The youngster may awaken and still meet the criterion, as long as he or she stays in the room and does not cause family disruption.

Comment

Ideally, we recommend that the youngster sleep alone for 1 week. Recognizing that working with a child or adolescent with WCE will be more challenging and time consuming, consent will depend on a family's willingness and/or ability to accomplish these goals. You may have to compromise your expectations and help families realize a reasonable degree of success, given the specific circumstances. In Chapter 9 we demonstrate how child, parent, and family factors interact during the treatment process.

DEALING WITH ACTUAL PHYSICAL ILLNESS

Unlike most youngsters who rarely experience their physical fears (e.g., vomiting, choking, fainting), Montana's fear of vomiting was grounded in reality. Given her reflux condition, moderate levels of anxiety were enough to trigger vomiting episodes. The slightest physical sensation caused her to become hysterical, prompting the need to be nearby her mother. As a result, we need to target the frequency of her vomiting episodes as well as her FBA.

Fear of Physical Illness versus Actual Physical Illness

Youngsters who fear being alone/sleeping alone due to FPI need a safe person nearby just in case they get sick. Given that the youngster rarely (if ever) experiences the feared outcome, the fear remains abstract and ubiquitous. Thus, the focus of treatment is showing (through exposure) the youngster that his or her feared outcome is unlikely and, indeed, manageable.

Youngsters who experience actual physical illness (API), however, tend to be afraid only to the extent that the actual illness continues to occur. Treating API is more about dealing with a tangible outcome than an abstract fear. As a result, the focus of treatment is to minimize or eliminate the API. Typically youngsters with API-induced separation anxiety have a physical condition (e.g., reflux, asthma, enuresis/encopresis) as well as anxiety.

Parenting Styles and Sleeping Alone

Mrs. M. (overprotective indulgent) spent an inordinate amount of time with Michael at night for fear of causing him further distress. Mrs. P. (overprotective controlling) stayed with Brian as long as necessary but resented his resistance to sleeping in his own room at night. Mrs. W. was neither indulgent nor intrusive. In fact, she was able to set limits with Montana in a supportive way. If anything, Mrs. W. may have initially spent *too little* time with Montana. For example, she would stay with Montana at night, but often leave before she fell asleep. If Montana awakened at night and came into her parents' bedroom, Mrs. W. would immediately bring her back to her own bedroom. Again, Mrs. W. would often leave before Montana fell asleep. This pattern was surprising, given that Montana was experiencing frequent vomiting episodes. It may have stemmed from Mrs. W.'s desire to help her daughter "handle" her fears. Although admirable and executed with good intentions, the frequency of Montana's vomiting episodes necessitated a modification to the nighttime routine.

Treatment Planning

API Plan

STEP 1: BREAK THE CYCLE

First of all, and most importantly, we need to break the cycle of Montana's vomiting episodes and reestablish a safety zone. In order to do this, Mrs. W. needs to stay with Montana (in Montana's bedroom) until she falls asleep. Similarly, if Montana awakens and comes to her parents' bedroom, Mrs. W. should return her daughter to her room and stay with her until she falls asleep. This approach appears to be a step backward, given Mrs. W.'s facility with Steps 1 (Back to the Bedroom) and 2 (The Phase Out). But it's a small concession if it helps to minimize Montana's vomiting episodes.

Criterion

One to two vomiting episodes per week.

Comment

Given the newly established safety zone, minimal anxiety is likely to occur. Most youngsters will reach this goal within 1 week. Now you can proceed with the remaining steps of the nighttime routine as long as you maintain the youngster's perception of control.

STEP 2: THE PHASE OUT

Youngsters with API are less likely to resist the hallway scenario. Distance from a parent has minimal bearing unless strong fear is present. Nevertheless, we recommend proceeding with this step to further strengthen the safety zone (i.e., more time without vomiting episodes).

Criterion

No to one vomiting episode per week.

Comment

This goal is likely to be accomplished within 1 week. At this point, a youngster's confidence should be sufficient to attempt the next step.

STEP 3: ASSUME NORMAL NIGHTTIME ROUTINE

Naturally, you can expect some resistance here. In Chapter 9, Mrs. W. will use some modified coping exercises to help her daughter stay calm in her room without vomiting.

Criterion

The youngster experiences physical sensations, stays in room, and does not vomit on at least three separate occasions.

Comment

Notice that we did not simply set the criterion of 1 week free of vomiting episodes. It's quite possible that Montana could sleep through the night for 1 week. If so, we would not have a way of gauging whether or not Montana could successfully cope with the experience of the unpleasant physical sensations.

FEAR OF ABANDONMENT

Hierarchy Development

Natalie's Abandonment Fears

Youngsters who fear being abandoned generally cope well during an activity or situation as long as their safety signals are in place. It is the anticipation of being dropped off (abandoned) and the fear of not getting picked up that fuel the separation anxiety. Natalie's hierarchy items (see Figure 8.3) are representative of the kinds of separation-related fears you are likely to encounter in youngsters with FAb.

Modifying the Safety Signals

Once again, the context of the exposure and the presence/strength of the safety signal(s) will determine both the degree of separation anxiety and a youngster's willingness to be exposed. For example, exposures may be more or less anxiety provoking by varying

- Length of time
- Choice of safety signals
- Proximity/visibility of safety signal
- Planned (therapist assigned) versus spontaneous (naturally occurring) exposures
- Familiar versus unfamiliar persons/places/situations
- Vague (provide minimal information) versus specific (provide maximal details)
- Promises versus reasonable efforts (no guarantee)

Item	
	Less Fearful
School/camp	
Going to school or camp (without afternoon phone call to Mrs. C.)	
Going to school or camp (without Mrs. C. staying for 10 minutes)	
Taking the bus to school or camp	
Going to school in a carpool	
Getting picked up late	
Social/extracurricular	
Dance class	
Play dates	
Parties	
Going to an activity in a carpool	
Getting picked up late	
New babysitter	
Sleep-overs	
	More Fearful

FIGURE 8.3. Fear of being abandoned: Natalie's hierarchy items.

Comment

At intake, most youngsters may not appear to be experiencing acute school refusal behavior because of the mandatory nature of school attendance. As a result, parents are more likely to accommodate a youngster's choice of safety signals. In Natalie's case, Mrs. C. drove her to school and promised to stay home during the day as well as pick her up *on time* after school. The true nature of a youngster's separation-related school refusal behavior is revealed as you gradually remove his or her safety signals (see Chapter 10).

The decision to expose youngsters to less mandatory situations (e.g., play dates, parties) will depend on the caregiver's parenting style. Overprotective indulgent parents such as Mrs. M., for example, may be less likely to attempt exposures because they are afraid to cause their youngster distress. In contrast, overprotective controlling parents such as Mrs. P. and Mrs. C. will be more forceful in attempting exposures. The parent's success (and persistence) is likely to be a function of the youngster's degree of resistance. Thus, when designing your treatment program, it is helpful to pay attention to avoidance behaviors and the function of a youngster's safety signals. In the next section, we discuss our three-step plan to help youngsters manage their FAb.

Treatment Planning

STEP 1: THE FAMILIAR

First, let's target some familiar situations: Those scenarios in which the youngster has participated in the past but is now reluctant to attempt. A good starting point is a neighborhood activity (e.g., play date). The youngster usually is reluctant to go *unless* the primary caregiver agrees to specific promises so the youngster will feel safe (e.g., stay with the youngster the entire time, stay home, pick up the youngster on time).

For each first exposure (specific activity), the goal is to give the youngster the perception of control. As long as he or she is willing to attempt the exposure, you can continue to provide his or her choice of safety signals. This choice typically means that a parent stays at the event for the entire time. Remember, a willingness to be exposed (even with safety signals) is much better than complete avoidance. A few exposures conducted in this fashion build momentum for future exposures in which safety signals can be minimized successfully.

Criterion

An activity is completed with minimal (or no) use of safety signals; for example, being dropped off at a play date or after-school activity. It is best to use your judgment here. Some youngsters may need time to warm up (e.g., parent stays for 5 minutes) to an activity and/or require a built-in safety signal (e.g., emergency phone call, if needed) before separation occurs. As each exposure is successfully completed, continue to attempt more challenging scenarios from the hierarchy.

Comment

As you continue emphasizing familiar situations, you will also want to gradually modify and then eliminate some of the youngster's safety signals to make the exposures more difficult. Naturally, there is room for negotiation as long as the youngster continues to maintain a perception of control.

STEP 2: THE UNFAMILIAR

Now we are entering unknown territory. Novel situations (e.g., play dates with new friends, parties) will be extremely anxiety provoking for youngsters who fear abandonment. Resistance is likely to be strong, especially for youngsters with strong-willed, high-intensity temperaments.

For each new exposure (specific activity), continue to allow the youngster to choose his or her safety signals. Conducting a few exposures in this fashion helps to build momentum. If resistance is strong, it may be necessary to repeat some previous exposures.

Criterion

An activity is completed with minimal (or no) use of safety signals. Again, be sure to respect a youngster's need for warm-up time and/or the need for a built-in (emergency) safety signal. You can then work your way through the hierarchy so at least a representative sample of situations has been addressed.

Comment

As with Step 1, if you modify or eliminate some of the safety signals, the exposures will be more difficult. Again, there is room for negotiation, keeping in mind the need to maintain a youngster's perception of some degree of control. The application of prescriptive coping skills and/or rewards is of vital importance here. A youngster's resistance is likely to be strong. You may need to start with one specific exposure and gradually weaken the strength of the youngster's choice of safety signals over time. Be sure to focus on a youngster's efforts (i.e., partial successes), rather than length of exposure and/or degree of anxiety experienced.

Clinical Tip

To help ensure success when attempting difficult exposures (highest items on the hierarchy), consider conducting transitional exposures as a first step. For example, sleep-overs are often extremely anxiety provoking simply due to the *length of time* a youngster is away from home. A youngster is more likely to succeed at staying with a close relative (safety signal) or neighborhood friend (safety signal) *before* attending a sleep-over further away from home—especially if the youngster engaged in sleep-overs in the past. The planned and more familiar sleep-over (which is still difficult) builds confidence for attempting any naturally occurring sleep-overs in the future. When they do occur, consider allowing some form of a safety signal (e.g., emergency phone call) to enhance the youngster's perception of control and increase the likelihood of success.

STEP 3: THE UNEXPECTED

At this point, you will have covered the bulk of the hierarchy items. Now conduct similar scenarios in which you increase separation anxiety by being *vague* about the details of the exposure and/or by encouraging *spontaneous* separations. Essentially, these modifications will seriously diminish the youngster's perception of control. In addition, you should encourage *unexpected* outcomes (e.g., parental lateness). In Chapter 10 we show you how to prepare youngsters for these scenarios, which constitute the strongest test of the power of prescriptive coping skills.

Worry about Calamitous Events versus Fear of Physical Injury

FAb/WCE (e.g., Natalie) tends to be associated with an insecure attachment to a primary caregiver; the youngster's fears are focused on the welfare of the caregiver. As a result, the caregiver willingly (overprotective indulgent) or reluctantly (overprotective controlling) accommodates the youngster's system of safety signals, thereby unwittingly promoting a false sense of security to short-circuit potential emotional outbursts. Typically, other family members fail to appease the youngster to a similar degree.

Alternatively, when FAb is maintained by FPI (e.g., Felicia), the youngsters' fears are focused on themselves; they fear venturing from home to avoid the possibility of becoming physically ill without having support nearby. This form of separation anxiety is not about an attachment to a primary caregiver. Thus, the youngster's system of safety signals typically includes a larger range of individuals (e.g., parents, siblings, relatives, friends, teachers, coaches, school nurse) who could provide the necessary aid, if needed.

FEARS OF BEING ALONE AND OF ABANDONMENT

Hierarchy Development

Felicia's Fears of Being Alone and of Being Abandoned

Brian and Michael both feared being alone during the day and/or night. In their cases, family members were always present *somewhere* in the house. Felicia, however, is afraid to *stay home alone*. This fear is more typical for adolescents, especially if their earlier FBA fears were never addressed. In addition, it would not be appropriate for parents to leave younger children home alone.

Older children and adolescents may not have a choice. At some point, they will be required to stay home alone. Parents are less likely to support FBA fears during this developmental stage. Felicia quickly learned to adapt to being home alone during the day, when both of her parents work. She always left the television or radio on to create the illusion that she was not alone. At night, however, was a different story. She dreaded seeing her parents go out, but she willingly let them go. Let's take a look at Felicia's FBA hierarchy items in Figure 8.4.

Modifying the Safety Signals: Fear of Being Alone

Once again, you can modify any of the safety signals associated with FBA to make a youngster's exposures more or less anxiety provoking:

- Length of time
- Choice of safety signals
- Proximity of safety signals
- Time of day
- Distance from home

Comment

The structure for targeting Felicia's fear of staying home alone should resemble the structure used for Brian's daytime fears. The process of moving through the hierarchy will be a little easier here, given Felicia's

Item	
	Less Fearful
Day	
Home alone (without radio or television)	
Parents take a walk	
Parents visit neighbor	
Parents run an errand	
Night	
Parents go out to dinner	
Sleep in attic (finished)	
	More Fearful

FIGURE 8.4. Fear of staying home alone: Felicia's hierarchy items.

behaviorally inhibited temperament. She was apprehensive about exposures but did not forcefully resist them. Rather, she exhibited more passive forms of resistance (e.g., watching television in parents' bedroom, unnecessary use of her bronchial inhaler). In addition, Felicia's parents were supportive and sensible: They recognized her anxiety but were not overly concerned about her losing her breath or vomiting.

Data suggested that neither parent was in need of parent training. Their chief roles during treatment would be to assist in setting up the exposures. Because both parents worked full time, they were content to spend free time at home; as a result, Felicia became too comfortable with their presence. At this point Felicia's parents were willing to socialize more so that Felicia could learn to be home alone without fear.

The bulk of Felicia's separation-related fears stemmed from her fear of abandonment. Let's take a look at Felicia's FAb hierarchy items in Figure 8.5.

Modifying the Safety Signals: Fear of Abandonment

For many adolescents, access to cell phones may be added to the list. Specific to Felicia is access to use of her bronchial inhaler. Children and adolescents with strong forms of FPI may utilize a number of personal objects as safety signals (e.g., water bottle). The standard safety signals for FAb can be modified in the following ways to make exposures more challenging:

- Length of time
- Choice of safety signals
- Proximity of safety signals (distance from home, bathroom)

Item	
	Less Fearful
School cafeteria	
Restaurants	
School-related sporting event (as spectator)	
Professional sporting event	
Car trips	
Sleepaway camp	
	More Fearful

FIGURE 8.5. Fear of being abandoned: Felicia's hierarchy items.

- Visibility of safety signals
- Familiar versus unfamiliar
- Access to cell phone and/or medical aid (e.g., bronchial inhaler)

Comment

The structure of targeting Felicia's FAb should resemble the approach taken with Natalie's abandonment fears (i.e., from familiar to unfamiliar to unexpected). Once again, the process of moving through the hierarchy will be a little easier, given Felicia's behaviorally inhibited temperament. It will be important to pay attention to, and gradually eliminate, her passive forms of resistance during exposures (see Chapter 10). We want her progress to reflect newly acquired coping skills rather than her ability to circumvent difficult scenarios.

Targeting Interoceptive Avoidance

In Felicia's case, it will be important to target a fourth step as well involving situations in which physical avoidance is unacceptable. We are referring to her participation in track sports. Felicia *held back* in her participation for fear of vomiting or losing her breath. She needed to learn that she could exert herself and still regulate her breathing without use of her inhaler. Felicia always had someone close by as well as access to her cell phone and bronchial inhaler. She regularly used her inhaler before beginning her workouts. Her physician, track coach, and parents concurred that Felicia's preasthmatic condition did not necessitate the use of an inhaler. Felicia was told by all parties (i.e., physician, coach, parents) that she was physically able to run and was not at risk for developing any medical complications. Felicia and her parents very much wanted her to overcome her fears so that she could reach her full potential. Permission was granted for Felicia to participate in our program.

Intellectually, Felicia knew she was not at risk when running track, but despite repeated assurances from her physician and parents that an inhaler was unnecessary, she refused to run without it. Figure 8.6 shows the situations we targeted.

Modifying the Safety Signals

There are four different levels of safety signals that we can modify to help Felicia cope more effectively.

- Setting (home, gym, schools [home, away], neighborhood)
- Proximity of persons (parent, personal trainer, coach, friend)

Item	
	Less Fearful
Treadmill (home)	
Treadmill (gym)	
Track practice	
Running in neighborhood	
Track meet	
	More Fearful

FIGURE 8.6. Interoceptive avoidance: Felicia's hierarchy items.

- Degree of physical exertion
- Presence/absence/use of inhaler and/or cell phone

In Chapter 10 we show how we helped Felicia gradually eliminate these safety signals and negotiate her interoceptive avoidance.

WHAT'S NEXT?

In the next chapter we describe the process of negotiating a fear of being alone and/or sleeping alone in a step-by-step fashion for Brian, Michael, Montana, and their families.

CHAPTER 9

Negotiating Fear of Being Alone

Being Alone and Sleeping Alone

> If I go to [tennis] practice, an intruder will be [at home] robbing us.
> If I stay home [with my family], I will be safe.
>
> —MICHAEL

FEAR OF BEING ALONE DURING THE DAY AND AT NIGHT

At intake, Brian was terrified of being alone during the day and at night. His FPI largely maintained his FBA. During the day, Brian needed to be with someone at all times. His older sisters referred to him as "the shadow." At night, he would fall asleep on the couch in the family room with his father (Mr. P.). Any effort on his mother's part (Mrs. P.) to get Brian to sleep in his own room, alone, resulted in explosive outbursts that kept the entire family up for hours. Given Brian's insecure attachment and behaviorally uninhibited temperament, its high-intensity–slow-adaptability aspects, forceful resistance, and overt avoidance were expected. In the next section, we discuss the process of negotiating Brian's FBA in a step-by-step fashion.

Negotiating the Daytime Routine

In Brian's case, we began the process of exposure by encouraging him to play in his bedroom alone. In Dialogue 9.1 we illustrate how we negotiated the first exposure and sealed the deal with a contingency contract.

Dialogue 9.1

THERAPIST: Are you ready to try and play in your room alone?

BRIAN: (*Starts to cry, breathes heavily.*)

THERAPIST: Let's take a deep breath. (*Demonstrates.*)

BRIAN: (*Takes a deep breath.*) I can't.

THERAPIST: Let's practice the exercises (*demonstrates.*)

BRIAN: (*Practices.*)

THERAPIST: Good. Are you calm?

BRIAN: (*Nods weakly.*)

THERAPIST: What would make it easier for you to stay in your room?

BRIAN: (*Shrugs shoulders.*)

THERAPIST: Would it help if your door was left open?

BRIAN: (*Nods, offers half smile.*)

THERAPIST: What else?

BRIAN: See my mom.

Negotiate

THERAPIST:
How about if you could *hear* your mom.

BRIAN: (*Starts to get teary.*)

THERAPIST: She could stay in the hallway by the bathroom.

BRIAN: Could I talk to her?

THERAPIST: You could ask her one question.

BRIAN: (*Starts to cry again.*) I can't . . .

THERAPIST: Brian, I know it's hard, and it's okay if you get scared. But the only way you will overcome being scared is to let yourself get scared. You have to show yourself that nothing bad will happen to you.

BRIAN: I *can't* . . .

THERAPIST: Tell me it's hard, but you'll try.

BRIAN: It's too hard!

Reward

THERAPIST: What reward would you like to work for? (*Looks at rewards list.*)

BRIAN: (*Quickly calms down.*) A pack of cards?

Minimum and Maximum Goals

THERAPIST: Could you stay in your room for 5 minutes?

BRIAN: That's too long.

THERAPIST: How about at least 2 minutes, but you try and stay for 5 minutes?

BRIAN: (*Nods.*)

THERAPIST: If you get scared, what will you do?

BRIAN: Practice my exercises.

THERAPIST: Show me.

BRIAN: (*Performs relaxation exercises with fists, jaw, shoulders, stomach.*)

THERAPIST: Good.

Contract

THERAPIST: Let's fill in the contract together (see Chapter 7).

Parent Education

It's important to help parents understand what to expect during the first exposure. We prepared Mr. and Mrs. P. to expect any of the following behaviors from Brian:

- Refuses to stay in room.
- Leaves room prematurely.
- Cries or whines.
- Explodes into tantrum.
- Unleashes personal attacks (e.g., "I hate you" or "You don't love me").

In addition, you can help parents understand that most oppositional behaviors are a function of a youngster's temperament, attachment, and anxiety sensitivity. Such behaviors are best viewed as a youngster's desperate efforts to avoid separation-anxious situations, rather than any form of intrinsic manipulation.

Parent Skills

We find it helpful to review and discuss the following strategies to help ensure that parents effectively implement the exposure.

- Reinforcing partial successes.
- Implementing the VRI approach: *V* (validate), *R* (remind of reward/practice coping skills), *I* (ignore).
- Utilizing existing behaviors by shaping them.

In Dialogue 9.2, we discuss these parent strategies with Mr. and Mrs. P.

Dialogue 9.2

THERAPIST: Remember, any demonstration of effort on Brian's part is a success and worthy of praise. Your goal is to help him stay in his room for as long as he can and to use the relaxation exercises to "take away" his anxiety rather than your presence. Do your best to keep him from seeing you. You may have to talk him through the exposure more than you would prefer. Use the VRI acronym. For example:

V: "I know you're scared, and it's okay to be scared."
R: "Practice your breathing and relaxation exercises and think about getting your cards."

After the first two steps, do your best to *I*gnore his fearful displays (i.e., whining, crying, yelling). Periodically, you may have to say, "I cannot talk to you until you're calm." This way you would be reinforcing his calming rather than fearful behaviors. If necessary, reinforce Brian's coping behaviors (i.e., practicing exercises, acting appropriately) by offering periodic praise prompts, such as "You're doing great," to keep him on task. If he steps out of his room, gently encourage him to go back. Consider trying this exposure at least once a day until he meets the 2-minute criterion.

MR. P.: A pack of cards for staying in his room for 2 minutes? It seems like a little much.

THERAPIST: I understand your concern (*addressing Mr. P.*). As Brian makes progress, we'll phase out the tangible rewards. It often helps to start with a more potent reward to build momentum.

MRS. P.: I'll do whatever helps. It's only a few dollars.

THERAPIST: I need you both to sign the contract.

MRS. P.: (*Looks over quickly, then signs.*)

MR. P.: (*Looks over carefully, sighs, then signs.*)

Brian stayed in his bedroom for 3 minutes. However, he stood at the edge of his door and repeatedly peeked out so that he could see his mother. Mrs. P. tried the VRI acronym but became frustrated after several times and yelled for Brian to get in his room. Brian complied but kept calling out that he had to go to the bathroom. As Brian escalated, Mrs. P. relented at the 3-minute point to let Brian go to the bathroom. Mr. P. and Mrs. P. were at odds about whether or not Brian should receive his reward.

Therapist Decision

Brian should receive his reward. He *did stay* in his room for 3 minutes. Given that it was the first assignment and resistance was expected, he did better than anticipated. As you can imagine, Mr. P. was not thrilled by this decision. Mrs. P. was upset because she believed that her husband should have no say in the matter, given that he was not present during the exposure. We validated both parents' points of view. For example, Mrs. P. was correct in her decision to reward Brian. Mr. P.'s concerns were validated in the sense that Brian "cheated" during the exposure. In the spirit of moving forward, we convinced Mr. P to agree to reward Brian. However, we explained to Brian that he would need to complete several similar assignments *without cheating* before receiving the next reward.

Clinical Tip

Remember that it is important to reward to a criterion. Once the youngster receives a reward for a specific exposure, you will need to create the expectation that he or she will no longer receive a reward for a similar exposure. The task is now viewed as part of his or her repertoire.

The bedroom exposure was repeated two times until Brian could stay alone for 5 minutes without cheating. Several similar exposures (e.g., in the family room, kitchen, bathroom) of equal length were assigned. However, Mrs. P. was now positioned further away (but on the same floor) so that Brian could not see or hear her. Brian stayed in his room but still continued to call out or request to go to the bathroom. This time, however, Mrs. P. used the VRI acronym once and waited until the 5-minute interval was up.

In the next reward-based exposure Brian was required to stay alone in the family room for 30 minutes; he was encouraged to practice his exercises and watch a favorite television show. His older sister (12 years old) would remain on the same floor, and his mom would be upstairs. Brian would receive a small Lego set for his efforts.

Brian had minimal difficulty completing the exposure. Distraction (from the television program) diluted both his sense of time and separation anxiety. Brian realized that he *could* stay alone for 30 minutes. As a result, he was *now willing* to attempt less distracting exposures (e.g., staying alone in his room). Following the success of staying in his room alone for 30 minutes, Brian was ready for the next part of the program.

Comment

During the previous sequence of exposures, Brian's perception of control was maintained by having a family member present on the same floor. Now it was time for Brian to stay alone on a *different* floor. Psychologically, this step challenges a youngster's perception of control and is likely to trigger a healthy amount of resistance. In Dialogue 9.3, we prepare Brian for the inevitable.

Dialogue 9.3

THERAPIST: Brian, you stayed in your room for 30 minutes?

BRIAN: (*Smiles.*) I did.

THERAPIST: That's great! How'd you do that?

BRIAN: I don't know.

THERAPIST: Did you practice your [relaxation] exercises?

BRIAN: (*Nods.*)

THERAPIST: Great! I'll bet you can do anything now.

BRIAN: (*Half-smile, shrugs his shoulders.*)

THERAPIST: Could you stay in your room while everyone else is downstairs?

BRIAN: (*Starts to cry.*) No . . .

THERAPIST: Brian . . .

BRIAN: I can't . . .

THERAPIST: Let's take a deep breath.

BRIAN: My stomach hurts. I want my mom. (*Gets up, reaches for the door.*)

THERAPIST: Brian, please come back. Let's figure this out.

BRIAN: (*Turns around, continues to cry.*)

THERAPIST: Brian, please sit down.

BRIAN: (*Sits down, holds his stomach.*)

THERAPIST: Will you take a deep breath with me?

BRIAN: (*Nods, starts to breathe.*)

THERAPIST: Good. Let's practice the stomach exercise. (*Demonstrates.*)

BRIAN: (*Tenses his stomach hard, then relaxes.*)

THERAPIST: Again. (*Both tense and relax.*)

BRIAN: (*Sighs with relief.*)

THERAPIST: Feel better?

BRIAN: (*Nods his head.*)

THERAPIST: Good. Did you *really* stay in your room for 30 minutes?

BRIAN: (*Nods weakly.*)

THERAPIST: How about you watch TV with your family, then go upstairs to get your mom her slippers?

BRIAN: (*Shrugs shoulders.*)

THERAPIST: Are you fast?

BRIAN: (*Smiles.*)

THERAPIST: How long would it take you?

BRIAN: Five seconds.

THERAPIST: Are you *The Flash*?

BRIAN: Yes.

THERAPIST: Reward?

BRIAN: A Bioncle (*small size*).

THERAPIST: Do we have a deal?

BRIAN: (*Smiles.*)

Parent Education

We think you'll find that not every parent understands the significance of the upstairs/downstairs exposure. It's no longer simply about the *amount of time*. If it were, clearly 30 minutes alone in a room is more difficult than 5 seconds. It is important to help parents understand the psychological impact (i.e., greater loss of control) of the upstairs/downstairs exposure. Here again you create the expectation for resistance and prepare the parent to address it.

As could be expected, Brian initially resisted during the exposure. Mrs. P. reminded Brian that *any* effort would be a *good* effort. In addition, she implemented the VRI acronym, but to no avail. Brian continued to make excuses that he "wasn't ready" and that he needed just "5 more minutes" of the television show. A frustrated Mrs. P. then asked her husband to get involved. As a result, Mr. P. stood up (from the couch), raised his voice, and walked with Brian to the edge of the staircase. Brian cried hysterically and refused to let go of the banister. After about 1 minute, Mr. P. walked back to the couch and resumed watching his television show. Mrs. P. then walked over to Brian and promised to watch him go up the stairs. Brian calmed down, then raced up the stairs to get his mom's slippers.

Comment

The exposure was a success and did a great deal for enhancing Brian's confidence to be alone. As you can see, however, some improvisation was necessary to help maintain Brian's perception of control in the face of resistance. Both parents became frustrated. The difference, however, was that Mrs. P. persisted because she was genuinely interested in helping her son. Mr. P. was simply "going through the motions." He appeared more concerned about missing his television show than helping his son negotiate separation anxiety. In cases like this, the degree to which parents follow through often determines treatment outcome.

At this point, Brian was ready to attempt the basement exposure. For years, Brian had refused to spend any time in the basement. The basement was recently finished, and his parents were beginning to resent his refusal to play down there. In fact, he was reluctant to play with his friends there as well. We maintained Brian's perception of control with the following sequence of exposures:

- Basement with both sisters (30 minutes)
- Basement with one sister (30 minutes)
- Basement alone (30 minutes)

The first two exposures were designed to increase Brian's comfort/familiarity with the basement. Of course, he had no concerns. The third and most important exposure was assigned as a *super exposure*. For example, Brian had to spend a minimum of 5 minutes a day in the basement alone (consecutively) until he reached the 30-minute criterion. The *minimum* of 5 minutes maintained his perception of control. The goal was to increase the duration of time in the basement each day. He could accomplish his goal in one day or progress at his own pace, as long as he stayed down there each time for longer intervals. In addition, we modified the safety signals over time to gradually make the exposure more difficult (i.e., differing degrees of distraction).

As long as you maintain a youngster's perception of control, the above sequence of exposures should proceed relatively smoothly. Of course, the time frame may differ and is usually a function of the youngster's motivation, severity of FBA, and the family's ability to set limits.

Brian demonstrated some expected resistance during the first two exposures (e.g., reluctance to go downstairs, calling out, bathroom excuses), but Mrs. P. handled him aptly. Brian took 1 week to reach the criterion and was rewarded at the end of the week. The super exposure counted as one assignment. Brian was now ready to tackle the night-time routine.

Negotiating the Nighttime Routine

Brian had no difficulty falling asleep (i.e., 10–15 minutes) in his bedroom as long as one parent stayed with him until he fell asleep. Mrs. P. stayed five of seven nights. During this week, Brian awakened in the middle of the night on eight separate occasions. Each time, he raced into his parents' bedroom. Mrs. P. then brought him back to his room and stayed with him until he fell asleep again (i.e., 5–10 minutes). Toward the end of the week, Brian slept through the night—likely a function of his overwhelming fatigue.

Comment

Given that Brian met the initial criterion (no immediate awakening) on the first night, we encouraged his parents to gradually move their chair further away from his bed to set the stage for the next step. We also created the expectation that he was allowed to disrupt his parents' sleep up to one time a night. This way, Brian would have to decide during each awakening if his fear warranted a parental visit. We also encouraged Brian to stay in his room and, if necessary, signal (e.g., call out) for his parents to *visit him*.

Parent Factor

At the same time, we encouraged Mr. and Mrs. P. to be firm (without too much emotion) when Brian tried to disrupt their sleep more than once a night. The parents were encouraged to follow our suggested sequence, based on Brian's persistence. They would:

- Stay in bed and pretend to be asleep.
- Stay in bed and practice VRI acronym.
- Stay in bed and demand (but not yell) that Brian go back to his bedroom.

Essentially, you are trying to help parents set limits without giving too much attention to a youngster's fearful displays. Brian required all three levels. However, once Mr. P. awakened and raised his voice, Brian stayed in his room.

Shifting the Rewards Structure

We shifted Brian's rewards from primarily tangible to social in nature. For example, Brian's reward for sleeping through the night on three occasions (need not be consecutive) included a sleep-over with one or both sisters over the weekend. In addition, the criterion of *sleeping through the night* now accepted night wakings that did not disrupt any family member's sleep. Finally, to help encourage success, the *morning* (i.e., when allowed to visit parents) began at 6:30 A.M. rather than 7:00 A.M.

As could be expected, Brian exhibited some relatively passive forms of resistance (e.g., frequent "good nights," bathroom excuses) during the first two nights, then fell into a comfortable routine. During this week, Brian slept through the night on two occasions. All other nights, he awakened one time, stayed in his room, signaled his need, and waited for a parent to visit. He was encouraged to listen to his tape or perform some distracting activities (e.g., read, play), so that he could wait as long as possible before disrupting his parents' sleep.

At the end of the week, Brian awakened at 6:00 A.M. and was able to occupy himself until visiting his parents at 6:30 A.M. As a result, he earned a sleep-over with his sisters on the weekend. Brian was now ready to negotiate the next level.

Awakening in the middle of the night was no longer a dreaded experience. In addition, Brian had slept through the night on several occasions. For this reason, some parents of children with similar patterns may not understand or accept heightened resistance at this stage. But, remember, Brian has always had someone to help him *fall asleep*.

Parent Education

It is important to create the expectation for healthy amounts of resistance ranging from relatively passive forms (e.g., calling out, frequent "good nights," bathroom excuses) to explosive hysterics. The intensity of a youngster's resistance at this stage is usually a function of temperamental variation, anxiety sensitivity, and degree of FBA fears. If at all possible, parents should attempt to stay in bed and follow the previous response sequence. In most cases, however, at least temporarily, young-sters may need to be escorted back to their bedroom.

Following his bedtime routine, Brian frequently called out to his parents and insisted that he needed to go to the bathroom. Mrs. P. implemented the VRI acronym and waited for her son to settle down. Brian started to cry and complained of terrible stomachaches. Both parents did their best to ignore Brian's cries for help, but within min-utes, he appeared at their bedroom door. Their efforts to be firm (i.e., insisting that Brian return to his bedroom) proved futile. Brian stayed in the hallway and kept the entire family up for hours. As a result, Mrs. P. relented and stayed in the hallway until Brian fell asleep.

Overcoming Resistance

As a first step, following the bedtime routine encourage parents to con-duct a "Quick Check" (Schaefer & Petronko, 1987) of his or her young-ster after 30 minutes. The visit should be brief and contingent upon a minimal number of call-outs, bathroom excuses, or parental visits. Once again, the youngster is reinforced for staying calm. The idea is to gradually eliminate the youngster's fearful behaviors and the need for any parental visits. Most parents can live with checking on his or her youngster one time per night.

Because the Quick Check is not a satisfactory solution for every youngster, another strategy that we have found helpful in challenging entrenched scenarios is the use of a baby monitor. The youngster is now assured that a parent will be *listening* for any signs of disturbance throughout the night. At the same time, the youngster stays in his or her room and comes to realize that nothing bad will happen to him or her. Simply that a parent *could hear* what's going on is sufficient. Keep in mind, however, that the use of a baby monitor is not as likely to work for youngsters who have FBA maintained by WCE. *What if* a parent falls asleep? This worry will need to be addressed as we help Michael negoti-ate his fears.

Brian liked the idea of a baby monitor. The first few nights, follow-ing his bedtime routine, Brian called out to *test* the assurance he had received that a parent would be listening. Brian's parents agreed to respond (i.e., stay in room and call back, "I'm awake") to his call-outs up to three times per night.

During the first week, Brian fell asleep each night within 30 min-utes. When he awakened in the middle of the night on two occasions, his parents took turns responding to him. Brian then fell asleep within 5 minutes. After three successful nights (i.e., no call-outs or awakenings), Brian's parents were instructed to gradually stop responding to his call-outs. When Brian was able to fall back asleep without parental reassurance, use of the baby monitor was gradually phased out (i.e., every other night, every three nights).

Mr. and Mrs. P. were not interested in eliminating their son's less potent safety signals (e.g., nightlight, "blankie"). They were completely satisfied with Brian's progress, especially after his first full week without causing any disruption at night. We used the next few sessions to address relapse prevention and termination issues (see Chapter 11).

FEAR OF BEING ALONE AT NIGHT

At intake, Michael's separation anxiety was beginning to spill over to his after-school activities. For example, he was passively resisting tennis practice (i.e., he disliked taking the school bus) and insisted that his mother pick him up after school. Mrs. M. reported knowing that Michael was afraid to come home after dark. Given the neighborhood robbery and Michael's subsequent fears, she did not want to make his life "any more difficult." From our perspective, Michael's behaviorally inhibited temperament suggested strong passive resistance and covert avoidance as expected features. In the next section, we discuss the process of negotiating Michael's FBA in a step-by-step fashion.

Negotiating Nighttime Fears

The process of behavioral exposure began by having Michael attend tennis practice. As we illustrate in Dialogue 9.4, his reluctance stemmed from his *all-or-nothing thinking*.

Dialogue 9.4

THERAPIST: Are you going to tennis practice tomorrow?

MICHAEL: No (*looks down*).

THERAPIST: Your mom tells me you're the best one on the team.

MICHAEL: (*Looks up with a half-smile.*)

THERAPIST: Do you want to play?

MICHAEL: (*Nods.*)

THERAPIST: How could we make it easier for you?

MICHAEL: (*Shrugs shoulders.*)

The problem was that Michael was approaching the situation in all-or-nothing terms:

"If I go to [tennis] practice, an intruder will be [at home] robbing us."

"If I stay home [with my family], I will be safe."

Michael didn't realize that different options were available that could enhance his perception of control. We suggested the following:

- Attend part of the practice (come home before dark).
- Parent stays for part or all of practice session.
- Parent picks him up after practice (rather than using carpool or bus transportation).
- Parent agree to enter house first upon arrival.

Comment

Michael liked the idea of the first two options; simply knowing that the options were available enhanced his perception of control. However, to avoid any potential peer-related embarrassment, he chose the last two options. He was now willing to attend tennis practice. Because he had sufficient desire, a reward at this stage was not deemed necessary.

Parent Education

It was crucial that Mrs. M. know what to expect during this first exposure. Any resistance on Michael's part could have easily swayed her. As a result, we prepared Mrs. M. for any of the following behaviors from Michael:

- Reluctance or refusal to go to school (in the morning).
- Chooses not to attend practice (in the morning).
- Refusal to take bus home after school.
- Insists on being picked up before dark.
- Insists on parental promises (i.e., pick up after school, enter house first).
- Insists on calling during the day or before tennis practice.

Comment

The dynamic of working with a youngster such as Michael is quite different from working with someone such as Brian. For example, Brian is visibly fearful and resistant in session and at home. In some ways, his temperamental style is easier to address. The coping skills he learns in session will likely transfer to other settings.

Michael, however, is covertly (i.e., passive, withdrawn) fearful and resistant. His temperamental style *appears* to be more agreeable to treatment demands. As a result, at times, we are uncertain about what he is actually *willing* to do. Michael's passive nature also lends itself to "cheating" during exposures. For this reason, we pay greater attention to Michael's behavior (i.e., refusal to budge during exposures) than his emotions, and we keep in mind that Michael is just as intense and strong-willed as Brian. He simply shows it in a different way.

Parent Skills

We discussed the following strategies with Mrs. M., anticipating that she would have difficulty remaining firm and following through.

- Reinforcing partial successes.
- Implementing the VRI approach: *V* (validate), *R* (remind of reward/practice coping skills), *I* (ignore).
- Utilizing existing behaviors by shaping them.

As you can imagine, overprotective indulgent parents such as Mrs. M. have a difficult time with the *ignoring* part. For this reason, we needed to model *calm postures*. We demonstrated and explained how her fearful facial expressions and body language reinforced Michael's anxiety. We let her know that she could *think* whatever she feels, but that she should try to *show* her confidence in him through coping postures.

In addition, we needed to explain all possible scenarios that would constitute partial successes. For example, if necessary, it would be acceptable for Mrs. M. to attend the entire practice, but she would have to emphasize to Michael that he must do *something*, and that completely avoiding practice is not an option. The first exposure represents the beginning of effective limit setting.

As could be expected, Michael was reluctant to attend school. Rather than *give in* to his separation anxiety, as she had done previously, Mrs. M. discussed all of his options with her son. Michael requested to be picked up after practice (rather than taking the bus). In addition, he required promises from his mother to enter the house first and to have all the outside lights on. Michael also requested permission to call his mother during the day, if needed. In Dialogue 9.5 we helped Michael evaluate the exposure in a healthy way to build his momentum.

Dialogue 9.5

THERAPIST: How was tennis practice?

MICHAEL: Good.

THERAPIST: Did you get scared?

MICHAEL: (*Nods.*)

THERAPIST: What were your thoughts?

MICHAEL: Someone will be in the house.

THERAPIST: How did you handle those thoughts?

MICHAEL: Practiced (*my Stop.*) Had a sticker in my pocket.

THERAPIST: What were your other thoughts?

MICHAEL: I played before. I'll be okay.

THERAPIST: Good, but did you believe that?

MICHAEL: (*Shrugs his shoulders.*)

THERAPIST: Did your mom stay the entire time?

MICHAEL: She picked me up after [practice].

THERAPIST: Did you call her?

MICHAEL: No.

THERAPIST: That's great. What happened when you went home?

MICHAEL: (*Shrugs shoulders.*)

THERAPIST: Anyone waiting for you?

MICHAEL: No.

THERAPIST: What did you *show* yourself?

MICHAEL: Nothing bad happened?

THERAPIST: That's right. Just because you *think* someone will rob you, does that mean you will be robbed?

MICHAEL: No.

THERAPIST: So what should you say to yourself the next time you get scared?

MICHAEL: (*Shrugs shoulders.*)

THERAPIST: It's not me, it's my . . .

MICHAEL: Anxiety.

THERAPIST: Good. Did you praise yourself?

MICHAEL: Yes.

THERAPIST: Great. Will you go to the next practice?

MICHAEL: (*Nods.*)

THERAPIST: Can you take the bus or carpool home?

MICHAEL: (*Nods.*)

Michael was now expected to attend *all* after-school activities regularly. During each new exposure (i.e., different activity from tennis practice), we maintained his perception of control by initially allowing him to choose his safety signals. Once successful, we gradually modified the safety signals (e.g., required him to take bus or carpool, no emergency phone call) to make the exposures more difficult.

Michael had minimal difficulty completing the exposures. The initial tennis exposure was the catalyst, and within 2 weeks, Michael was attending all of his after-school activities. Along the way, we praised Mrs. M. for her newly developed ability to set limits with her son.

Comment

Like Brian, the upstairs/downstairs exposure served a similar purpose for Michael. However, there were notable differences. First, Michael's degree of fear was stronger. Second, Mrs. M. could not manage the same degree of resistance as Mr. and Mrs. P. Third, unlike Brian, Michael was not interested in spending time alone *at home*, because he truly believed that he was in danger. For these reasons, we set up the exposure so that Mrs. M. was positioned at the bottom of the stairs. We told Michael to run up quickly, retrieve an item, and run back down— with Mrs. M. in sight. We simply needed to show Michael that he *could* be alone *somewhere* in his house.

Michael was successful on the first attempt. Mrs. M. initiated the exposure and reassured Michael that she would remain at the bottom of the stairs. Several other similar exposures (i.e., super exposure) were then assigned until Michael could remain upstairs for 1 minute out of sight from his mother. When he reached the 1-minute criterion, he received a reward. At this point, for the first time, Mrs. M. was *hopeful* that Michael's separation anxiety could be eliminated. Michael was also pleased with his progress. It was time to move through the hierarchy.

Since the neighborhood robbery, Michael refused to be the first person to enter his house. However, that he was less anxious during the day because the robbery occurred at night. We maintained his perception of control with the following sequence of exposures:

- Enters house first (day); holds mother's hand.
- Enters house first (day); mother in sight.
- Enters house first (night); holds mother's hand.

- Enters house first (night); mother in sight, siblings upstairs.
- Enters house first (night); mother stays in garage, siblings upstairs.
- Enters house first (night); mother stays in garage, no one else home.

Comment

It may seem like a great number of exposures to conduct, but given that Michael was coming home several times a day, it was important to take advantage of these natural opportunities. This sequence of exposures should be assigned as a super exposure; psychologically, it is similar to the basement exposure for Brian. The one key difference is the time interval. Thirty minutes was deemed appropriate for Brian; given Michael's degree of fear, 1–2 minutes was more than adequate.

Of course, it's not surprising that Michael was most resistant during the last two exposures. When Mrs. M. stayed in the garage, Michael stuck his foot in the door. To help maintain his perception of control as the door was closed, his siblings stayed in the hallway (immediately visible), then the top of the stairs. During the final exposure, Michael talked to his mother through the garage door. Once successful, we repeated the exposure by having Michael perform his cognitive-based exercises out loud.

Negotiating the Nighttime Routine

Michael refused to go to sleep. He became so preoccupied about waking up alone that he remained uncomfortable even when his mother was present. As a result, he demanded that his mother promise to stay for the entire night. Despite her promises, he remained hypervigilant because he didn't trust that she would stay.

During the first week, Michael slept less than 2 hours per night. At times, when Mrs. M. fell asleep, Michael called out until she awakened. During the beginning of the second week, due to sheer fatigue, Michael started falling asleep within 2 hours. He did awaken, however, at least once per night to check to see if his mother was still there. After three consecutive nights of checking, his perception of control was enhanced, and he slept through the night.

Comment

The next step was to negotiate with Michael how long his mother would stay in his room at night. Michael accepted that it was taking him about

2 hours to fall asleep (data from Mrs. M.'s sleep log). We suggested that Mrs. M. initially stay for *4 hours*.

In session, Michael quietly agreed to allow his mother to leave. We knew otherwise, however, and prepared Mrs. M. for the inevitable (see Dialogue 9.6). Michael was encouraged to stay in his room, practice his cognitive-based exercises, distract himself, and if necessary, call for his mother to visit him.

Dialogue 9.6

THERAPIST: Michael is likely to be on guard again for most of the night, knowing that you will be leaving [after 4 hours].

MRS. M.: (*Sighs.*) I'm exhausted. I'm not sure how much longer I can go on. I can live with Michael falling asleep in 2 hours. I'll just bring my blanket and sleep on the floor.

THERAPIST: I know it's difficult, but you have to hang in there. If you give in to Michael now, all of your efforts will not be realized. He will have learned that persistence helps him to avoid separation anxiety.

MRS. M.: I know (*sighs*), but he *won't let me leave.*

THERAPIST: Could your husband help out?

MRS. M.: (*Laughs nervously.*) He gets up early [for work] in the morning. His sleep *cannot be disturbed.*

THERAPIST: Let's start over the weekend. How late does Michael typically stay up until?

MRS. M.: Ten o'clock.

THERAPIST: Would he have any objections if you allowed him to stay up later?

MRS. M.: (*Nervous laugh*) Not at all.

THERAPIST: Have Michael stay up until he can barely keep his eyes open. It will be very difficult for Michael to stay up, and if he does, his resistance will be much lower.

MRS. M.: Should I stay for 4 hours even if he falls asleep?

THERAPIST: Yes. The first two nights assure him that you will stay. Given his tiredness, 4 hours should be enough to help maintain his perception of control. Expect him to check that you are still there a few times. If he does, tell him, "I'm here."

MRS. M.: What if he wakes up and follows me into my room?

THERAPIST: Bring him back. Stand at the edge of his room and encourage him to practice his exercises. STOP stickers should be placed on the inside of his door and the outside of your door to cue his coping efforts. Use the VRI acronym. When he calms down, tell him you'll stand there until he falls asleep again. In this way, you are reinforcing him for *calming down* rather than becoming emotional when he enters your room. Each time he awakens, repeat this procedure.

Remember, it's okay if Michael becomes scared. We expect him to, and we made that clear to him. His reward is contingent on his *willingness* to comply with your commands.

MRS. M.: (*Nervous laugh*) I'll try. Wish me luck. (*Sighs.*)

The first night, as expected, Michael stayed up for 6 hours. Mrs. M. eventually fell asleep as well and stayed for the entire night. The second night, however, Michael fell asleep after 3 hours. He awakened two times to check that she was still there. Each time, Mrs. M. responded with "I'm here." At the fourth hour Mrs. M. returned to her bedroom, and Michael slept through the rest of the night.

To maintain Michael's perception of control during the phasing out of his mother as a safety signal, we disregarded the previous criterion of 4 hours. He was informed that as long as he *willingly* allowed his mother to stay in the hallway (i.e., sitting in a chair), she would initially stay there for the entire night.

During the first night, Michael couldn't settle down. He did not believe his mother would stay in the hallway. As a result, Mrs. M. was encouraged to keep her pillow and comforter (safety signals) in the hallway. By doing so, Michael was assured that she had no intention of returning to her bedroom.

For the next two nights, Michael was still on guard but to a lesser degree. He fell asleep after 4 and 3 hours, respectively. Each night he called out a number of times and periodically left his bed to check that his mother was still in the hallway. During the rest of the week, Michael fell asleep within 3 hours. Mrs. M. remained in the hallway for the entire night.

Comment

In session, we presented Michael with the data from Mrs. M.'s sleep log. He accepted that he had fallen asleep within 3 hours each night. He was beginning to appear more comfortable with the nighttime routine. He reported less fear regarding the possibility of an intruder robbing his house. His anxiety appeared more generalized in nature and stemmed from his inability to occupy himself at night when he awakened. We created the expectation that Mrs. M. would return to her bedroom after *4* hours (rather than three) to heighten his perception of control.

Parent Education

To facilitate negotiation of this step, we encouraged Mrs. M. to do the following:

- Begin over the weekend (encourage fatigue).
- Stand at edge of room during night wakings.
- Facilitate Michael's practice of cognitive-based exercises.
- Maintain less potent safety signals (keep Mrs. M.'s pillow or blanket in hallway after she returns to her bedroom).
- Enforce compliant-contingent rewards.

During the first night, Michael refused to fall asleep. Mrs. M. attempted to return to her bedroom after 4 hours, but Michael held onto her. She agreed to stand at the edge of his room until he fell asleep if he used his exercises to calm himself down.

When Michael fell asleep, Mrs. M. attempted to return to her bedroom. He yelled out twice (too tired to get up) for her to stay in the hallway. Due to fear that Michael would wake up her husband, Mrs. M. stayed in the hallway. Michael called out several more times during the night to be sure she was still there. Mrs. M. fell asleep in the hallway.

On the second night, exhausted, Michael fell asleep within 2 hours. Mrs. M. also fell asleep in the hallway. When she awakened in the middle of the night, she checked on Michael and then returned to her bedroom. Michael slept through the night. During the rest of the week, Michael had several more difficult nights. However, on two occasions he fell asleep within 1 hour and slept through the night. Mrs. M. stayed in her bedroom.

Michael was now ready to assume a normal nighttime routine. Mrs. M., however, was ready to give up, as can be seen in Dialogue 9.7.

Dialogue 9.7

MRS. M.: (*Eyes half closed, hunched posture*) I think it's time to take a break from the program. Michael slept through the night twice this week. I can live with staying in the hallway until he falls asleep. He's doing much better.

THERAPIST: I agree that Michael is doing better. And I know how hard you are working and *how tired* you are.

MRS. M.: (*Laughs weakly, then sighs.*)

THERAPIST: And it looks like Michael's fear (*of an intruder.*) is diminishing. He is beginning to realize that nothing bad is likely to happen. But Michael still has to learn how to occupy himself at night and to fall asleep on his own.

MRS. M.: He's always been a light sleeper.

THERAPIST: We still have some work to do. We're not quite there. I'd like to try one more strategy.

MRS. M.: (*Sighs.*)

Overcoming Resistance

One strategy that we have found helpful in challenging cases is the use of a walkie-talkie. By having two-way communication (unlike a baby monitor), youngsters can remain in their bedroom and still feel *in control* following a normal bedtime routine (i.e., still awake) and during night wakings. In addition to the use of a walkie-talkie, we helped both Michael and his mother develop *action plans*.

Michael's Plan

We helped Michael problem-solve (see Dialogue 5.8) by developing alternative actions to calling out, seeking reassurance, and visiting his mother. When awakened, he was encouraged to do the following *before* speaking to his mother on the walkie-talkie:

- Turn on bedroom light (safety signal).
- Turn on hallway light (safety signal).
- Practice self-control (STOP acronym) and cognitive therapy exercises.
- Employ distraction (read a book, get a glass of water).

Mrs. M.'s Plan

- Give brief reassurances ("I'm awake," "I hear you," "I'll listen for you").
- Encourage Michael's action plan.
- Go through STOP acronym.

In Dialogue 9.8 we prepare Mrs. M. for the following possible dialogue with Michael (via walkie-talkie).

Dialogue 9.8

MRS. M.: Why are you scared?

MICHAEL: I'm afraid.

MRS. M.: What are your bad thoughts?

MICHAEL: Someone's in the house.

MRS. M.: *Any evidence?*

MICHAEL: I don't know.

MRS. M.: What are your (other) good thoughts?

MICHAEL: No one's in the house.

MRS. M.: Have you stayed in your room before?

MICHAEL: Yes.

MRS. M.: Will you stay in your room?

MICHAEL: I'll try.

MRS. M.: *What is the most likely thing that could happen?*

MICHAEL: I'll be okay.

MRS. M.: Do you remember your reward?

MICHAEL: Yes.

MRS. M.: Read your book.

MICHAEL: Okay. Can I call you again?

MRS. M.: Use your exercises.

MICHAEL: Okay.

Clinical Tip

As a transition, if necessary, the parent can keep a chair in the hallway; the parent can also conduct Quick Checks. Eventually, however, you will phase out both safety signals while maintaining the youngster's perception of control.

During the first week, Michael stayed in his room the entire time each night. The added safety signals (i.e., bedroom and hallway lights) and the walkie-talkie helped maintain his perception of control. In essence, he was staying in his room *alone* and learning to fall asleep, albeit gradually. He was also learning how to occupy himself rather than to call upon his mother to take away his separation anxiety. The problem, however, was that Michael called his mother (for 1–2 minutes) each time he awakened. During the first week, he called her three to five times per night.

Comment

In session, we negotiated a deal that Michael was allowed to call Mrs. M. up to two times per night. If he stuck with that arrangement, he was allowed to keep both his room and hallway lights on, as needed. His reward, however, was contingent upon calling only one time per night. The second call was for emergencies and was used to enhance his perception of control.

During the second week, Michael used one call each night to help him fall asleep. Despite awakening more than once on most nights, he only called his mother one time. He was becoming increasingly comfortable staying in his room, practicing his exercises, and reading. One night Michael stayed up for 90 minutes without disrupting any family members. On two occasions, he slept through the night.

We continued to negotiate with Michael until he was allowed one emergency call, and the hallway light was no longer an option. During his best week, he slept through the night five times. He called his mother on two occasions, one of which he had a nightmare, and the other, he was feeling physically ill.

Given the challenges of this case, we did not approach Mrs. M. regarding any further treatment goals. She accepted Michael's use of the walkie-talkie as long as he kept it to a minimum. We used the last few sessions to address termination and relapse prevention issues (see Chapter 11).

FEAR OF BEING ALONE AND ACTUAL PHYSICAL ILLNESS

At intake, Montana was afraid to sleep alone at night. Upon awakening, she cried hysterically and then immediately vomited. Montana's FBA was maintained by actual physical illness (API). Given her young age, we worked with her mother (Mrs. W.) as a first step.

Negotiating the Nighttime Routine

Parent Skills

During the parent sessions, we discussed relaxation as both general anxiety-management and coping tools. The exercises required modification due to Montana's young age and limited abstract thinking abilities. Diaphragmatic breathing was implemented as follows:

Smell the flowers [breathe in] ... Blow out the candles [breathe out] ...

To make the breathing exercises salient, we provided Mrs. W. with pictures of youngsters performing both of these activities. She placed the pictures on the inside and the outside of Montana's bedroom door to cue her. In addition, we demonstrated several basic progressive relaxation exercises (e.g., fists, jaw, stomach) for Mrs. W. to teach and practice with Montana. A daily sticker chart (i.e., practice compliant) was constructed to encourage Montana's general practice of the relaxation-based exercises each night before bedtime.

Montana had no difficulty falling asleep (i.e., 10 to 15 minutes) in her bedroom as long as Mrs. W. stayed with her. During the week, Montana awakened in the middle of the night on five occasions. Each time, she raced to her parent's bedroom. Mrs. W. then brought her back to her room and stayed (i.e., sat in chair) until she fell asleep again (5 minutes). Montana did not experience any vomiting episodes during this week.

Despite the success of the first week, we proceeded with the phase-out process to further enhance Montana's perception of control. Mrs. W. was encouraged to spend less time in the hallway each night.

Montana had no difficulty falling asleep with Mrs. W. in the hallway. By the end of the week, she was falling asleep within 5 minutes. On three separate occasions, Montana visited her parent's bedroom. Mrs. W. brought her back to her room and stayed in the hallway. For the second straight week, Montana did not experience any vomiting episodes. Mrs. W. reported that, for the first time in a long while, Montana was her "sweet little self" again.

Shifting the Rewards Structure

Up to this point Montana was receiving rewards (i.e., stickers) for the general practice of her relaxation/breathing exercises. Now she was expected to stay in her room without the benefit of her most potent safety signal (i.e., Mrs. W.). Given her young age, it was difficult for her to appreciate the relevance of *staying in her room* without having access to her mother. As a result, we encouraged Mrs. W. to implement a grab-bag rewards system. Inexpensive items were wrapped and left for Montana at the edge of her room each night *after* she fell asleep. If she stayed in her room until morning (i.e., 7:00 A.M.), she was allowed to choose one grab-bag present.

Parent Education

We prepared Mrs. W. for what to expect as we approached a normal nighttime routine:

- Call-outs
- Bathroom excuses
- Stepping outside room/visiting parent's room
- Vomiting episodes

Parent Skills

Mrs. W. was encouraged to stay at the edge of her room and implement the VRI acronym.

> *V:* "I know you're scared."
> *R:* "Practice your breathing. If you stay in your room, you can choose a reward."

Based on the degree of Montana's fearful displays, Mrs. W. was instructed to:

- *I*gnore them.
- Make her attention contingent on Montana's practicing of the exercises.

If necessary, Mrs. W. was instructed to stand at the edge of Montana's room and facilitate the following sequence:

- Look/point to pictures (smelling flowers, blowing out candles).
- Model the breathing.
- Model the relaxation.

Comment

Montana had no difficulty falling asleep. She did awaken, however, three times during the week. During the first night's waking, Mrs. W. tried to facilitate Montana's coping from her own bedroom. Although Montana stayed at the edge of her room, she vomited.

On the second two occasions, Mrs. W. stood at the edge of Montana's room and helped her practice the exercises. Montana calmed down both times and took her grab-bag present to bed with her.

To further enhance Montana's perception of control, Mrs. W. was encouraged to facilitate Montana's coping from the edge of her daughter's room. During the second week, Montana awakened on two occasions but did not experience any vomiting episodes.

During the next 2 weeks, Montana awakened on two occasions but did not experience any vomiting episodes. The first time she went to the bathroom and did not disrupt any family members sleep; the second time, she responded to Mrs. W.'s encouragement (from her own bedroom) to stay in her room and practice her exercises.

Following this interval, rewards (stickers, grab-bag items) were phased out. Relapse prevention and termination issues were addressed (see Chapter 11) and booster sessions were scheduled.

WHAT'S NEXT?

In Chapter 10 we discuss the process of negotiating a fear of abandonment (FAb) in school, camp, and other settings for Natalie, Felicia, and their families.

Negotiating Fear of Being Abandoned

School, Camp, and Other Settings

I just want my life back. I'm tired. I cannot keep promising to stay home or tell her [Natalie] where I'm going . . . I need her [Natalie] to get over this.

—MRS. C.

FEAR OF ABANDONMENT

At intake, Natalie was apprehensive about being dropped off and picked up at school, parties, play dates, extracurricular activities, sleep-overs, and summer day camp. She refused to participate in activities unless her mother promised to stay and was visible for the entire time. Given Natalie's strong-willed temperament, insecure attachment, and WCE, forceful resistance and overt avoidance were expected.

Negotiating the Familiar in the School Setting

On the surface, it appeared that Natalie was experiencing minimal anxiety/avoidance *before and after* school. Keep in mind, however, that she had the following safety signals in place:

- Natalie called her mother from school every day before lunch.
- Mrs. C. promised to stay home during school hours or was very specific about her whereabouts.
- Mrs. C. drove Natalie to school every day and stayed in the hallway until she was settled in the classroom.

As a first step, we negotiated with Natalie to consider giving up her daily 11:30 A.M. phone call to her mother. This was a good place to start because Natalie reported minimal anxiety around the time of the phone calls. She did, however, find comfort from her mother's additional reassurances to pick her up after school.

Natalie refused to skip a phone call outright. To maintain her perception of control, we emphasized *partial successes* in the form of a super exposure. For example, her minimum goal was to wait 30 minutes longer each day to call her mother, until she eventually skipped her phone call. If she became anxious, she would practice her prescriptive cognitive-based exercises. We recommended for Natalie to keep a STOP sticker in her pocket to cue her coping abilities.

As you can imagine, Natalie was not thrilled with this idea, but given that she *could call*, she was willing to try. A reward, however, was contingent on skipping her daily phone call one time during the week. On her first attempt, Natalie's anxiety got the best of her. She did, however, wait for 5 minutes.

Parent Education

Our goal was to help Natalie become less dependent on her need to speak with her mother during the school day. As a result, we framed the phone calls as opportunities for Mrs. C. to facilitate Natalie's coping. We emphasized partial successes and expected resistance on Natalie's part, due to the threat of giving up her safety signals. We prepared Mrs. C. to expect the following behaviors from Natalie:

- Crying or whining
- Angry outbursts
- Personal attacks

Parent Skills

In Dialogue 10.1 (phone call from school), Mrs. C. facilitated Natalie's coping skills and began the process of becoming increasingly vague, regarding her plans or whereabouts.

Dialogue 10.1

MRS. C.: (*Answering the phone*) Hi, Natalie, are you having a good day?

NATALIE: Yes . . . promise me you'll pick me up on time?

MRS. C.: What do you think?

NATALIE: *Mom* . . .

MRS. C.: Practice your STOP.

NATALIE: *Mom* . . . I have to go. *Promise me.*

MRS. C.: What's your *good* [coping] thought?

NATALIE: I don't know (*angry tone*).

MRS. C.: *Natalie* . . .

NATALIE: You always pick me up (*softly*).

MRS. C.: I'll see you later . . .

NATALIE: *Mom* . . .

MRS. C.: You can do it. I have to go . . .

On her next attempt, Natalie waited for 1 hour before calling her mother. Although Mrs. C. praised her efforts, Natalie found her dialogue to be even *less* reassuring. As a result, Natalie focused her efforts on skipping the phone calls and earning a reward.

During the first week, Natalie refrained from calling Mrs. C. for 3 days. Given Natalie's enhanced confidence, the second (super) exposure was for 4 phone-free days, with a bonus reward for 5 days. Following her success, we created the expectation that phone calls were allowed on an emergency basis (i.e., physical illness), and that only school personnel could make a call (e.g., teacher, nurse, guidance counselor).

Comment

Mrs. C. was eager to facilitate Natalie's progress. She decided that Natalie no longer needed to know her specific whereabouts. Power struggles ensued, and an overwhelmed Natalie threatened to cease her participation in the program. In Dialogue 10.2 we validated Mrs. C.'s frustrations and helped her to stay focused on the treatment program's objectives.

Dialogue 10.2

THERAPIST: Natalie did great this week. She no longer needs to call you from school.

MRS. C.: I know . . . (*sighs.*) I just want my life back. I'm tired.

THERAPIST: I know it hasn't been easy for you. And you're working very hard to help her.

MRS. C.: (*Smiles weakly.*)

THERAPIST: But please understand that we cannot coerce Natalie to overcome her separation anxiety. We have to help her to progress at her own pace. As you know, she's strong-willed . . .

MRS. C.: (*Nervous laugh.*)

THERAPIST: If we push Natalie too hard too fast, she'll refuse to participate. With each exposure, we build momentum.

MRS. C.: Do I have to keep telling her where I am at all times?

THERAPIST: As a transition, you can tell her only that you will be *local* or *out of town.*

MRS. C.: I'll try anything!

The next series of exposures was designed to eliminate Mrs. C.'s presence at school after the morning drop-off. Natalie insisted that her mother remain in the hallway until she was settled (10 minutes). To maintain Natalie's perception of control during the following sequence of exposures, we modified her safety signals along the following parameters:

- Length of exposure: Mrs. C. in the hallway from 8 minutes to 1 minute.
- Proximity of Mrs. C.: From outside the classroom to outside the building to waiting in the parking lot.
- Use of safe person: Natalie enters building with a friend; Mrs. C. waits in the parking lot.
- Use of safe person: Natalie enters without a friend; teacher greets at entrance.
- Goal: Natalie enters alone, teacher greets in hallway (outside of classroom).

As could be expected, the first few exposures were difficult, because Natalie did not trust that her mother would remain in the hallway. As a result, we offered her one Quick Check each morning. After a few mornings, Natalie felt secure until it was time for Mrs. C. to step outside the building.

To maintain Natalie's perception of control, Mrs. C. agreed to initially *show herself* during Natalie's Quick Check. When it came time for Mrs. C. to wait in the parking lot, she promised to stay during the first two exposures. As Natalie became anxious, her teacher prompted her to practice the STOP (she had a sticker on her desk). If Natalie remained in the classroom, she was rewarded with a special privilege during the day.

The last series of exposures went relatively smoothly as we re-placed Mrs. C. with less potent school-based safety signals (safe per-sons). The use of individuals in the school setting helped to ensure the durability of Natalie's progress. Our next step was for *someone else* to take Natalie to school in the morning.

Comment

In our experience, when it comes to attending school, the majority of separation-anxious youngsters resemble Natalie. As long as the safety signals are in place, school attendance is typically adequate. The prob-lem, however, is that eventually parental or school-based accommoda-tions become overwhelming and cannot be maintained.

In Natalie's case, we were careful to maintain her perception of control at all times. In addition, we educated Mrs. C. and school per-sonnel about what to expect. Too often, separation-related school refusal behaviors are viewed as attention seeking and oppositional in nature. Such an interpretation may create a "therapeutic" process that is actually antagonistic and coercive. If we allowed Mrs. C. or school personnel to perceive Natalie in this way, she may have shut down and adamantly refused to participate. Some youngsters (around 8%; Kear-ney & Silverman, 1996) may meet the criteria for oppositional defiant disorder. Nevertheless, what's important to keep in mind are the func-tions of these challenging behaviors.

For example, when anxiety (separation, panic, worry) appears to be the predominant feature, externalizing symptoms (tantrums, freez-ing, verbal/physical outbursts) are likely to help youngsters ameliorate or avoid anxiety-provoking situations. Alternatively, when serious con-duct issues emerge (e.g., vandalism, truancy, drug use), more compre-hensive approaches are deemed necessary (see Kearney, 2001).

When Fear of Attending School Is Intense

For some youngsters, the fear of being abandoned is so intense that the morning routine is unbearable. In such cases you can expect any of the following behaviors:

- Explodes into tantrum.
- Refuses to get dressed.
- Refuses to eat.
- Aggresses verbally or physically.
- Locks self in bathroom.
- Clings to caregivers.

- Refuses to get out of car.
- Runs out the school building.

In Natalie's case, the safety signals were already in place. The idea was to eliminate them gradually and to replace them with prescriptive coping skills. In more intense scenarios, however, the process of exposure is likely to be more gradual, and the safety signals will need to be "built in" to encourage exposures. Remember, any effort toward experiencing exposure *even with safety signals* is better than complete avoidance. The steps in this more intense scenario may occur as follows:

- Child gets ready in the morning, with no expectation of going to school.
- Child sits in the car in the parking lot, with no expectation of entering school.
- Child walks into school with parent, then walks out.
- Child stays in the hallway with parent for specified amount of time.
- Child stays in nonacademic area with parent (e.g., library).
- Child stays in one class, with parent present or in the hallway.

This sequence is typical for youngsters in preschool through the elementary grades. Young children may have difficulty understanding the concept of exposure. In addition, they may also have a poor *sense of time*. As a result, *any* parental absence is likely to be perceived as extremely anxiety provoking. Remember, each step is negotiable as long as the youngster willingly attempts the exposures. Be sure to emphasize partial successes. If difficulty entering or staying in the school building (i.e., runs out) persists, consider the following suggestions:

- Use spontaneous rewards to unlock the separation-anxiety response pattern (e.g., trading cards, trinkets).
- Post familiar peer(s) or teacher(s) at entrance.
- Mention possible truancy offense (in a nonthreatening manner) as another means of helping youngsters enter and stay in the school building.

Once the above sequence of exposures is negotiated, most youngsters with FAb are open to having their parent phased out of the process. Even so, you may have to add other safety signals initially, such as:

- Parental promises to stay home
- Periodic phone calls
- Periodic parental visits (e.g., lunchtime)

In some cases, however, school-related FAb may entail changes in a larger context. For example, chaotic morning, daytime, and nighttime routines may need to be restructured to minimize distress and create more comfortable surroundings for the entire family. In addition, rewards and consequences may need to be negotiated based on the child's degree of compliance with these newly established routines.

In our experience, once youngsters with FAb get over the anticipatory hurdle (WCE) of attending school, the rest of the day typically goes smoothly, especially if safety signals are in place and only eliminated gradually.

When staying in school is the problem, other problems or disorders may be present. For example, somatic complaints (Stickney & Miltenberger, 1998), depressive symptoms (Kearney, Silverman, & Eisen, 1989; for a review, see Kearney, 1993), panic attacks (Hayward, Taylor, Blair-Greiner, & Strachowski, 1995), and social anxiety are often observed in older children and adolescents and associated with chronic school refusal behavior (for a full explication, see Kearney, 2001).

Negotiating the Familiar in Other Settings

As we move through the hierarchy, it's important to keep in mind that Natalie *was attending* school. Helping her to negotiate school-related situations was a matter of gradually removing her safety signals while preserving her perception of control. On the other hand, at intake, she was largely avoiding her social/extracurricular activities. With the exception of attending her dance class, she frequently turned down invitations for play dates, parties, or sleep-overs that were held in other youngster's houses. As a result, we expected greater resistance on her part, because most of her familiar situations were only vaguely familiar (i.e., her participation was sporadic).

Negotiating Natalie's dance class was similar to phasing out Mrs. C.'s presence in the school setting. The sequence of exposures was as follows:

- Mrs. C. steps out of viewing distance for 2–5 minutes (stays in building).
  Quick check if needed (phase out).
- Mrs. C. steps outside the building (promises to stay there for 2 minutes).
  Show yourself (Mrs. C.) if needed (phase out).

- Mrs. C. leaves the building (walks to get a drink nearby—5 minutes).
- Mrs. C. sits in car in the parking lot (10–15 minutes).
- Mrs. C. takes car to run errands (5–30 minutes).

Comment

The turning point is typically the first car-related exposure. Youngsters with WCE may fear that their parent will leave the parking lot. For example, Natalie refused to go to dance class unless Mrs. C. promised to leave her car keys in a locker. Naturally, this scenario could constitute a first step. However, sometimes youngsters refuse to take the next step. In Natalie's mind, she was finished with the program. In Dialogue 10.3, we reframed Natalie's frustrations and helped her to move forward.

Dialogue 10.3

NATALIE: Thank you for your help, but I won't be coming anymore.

THERAPIST: Why not?

NATALIE: I don't need too, that's all.

THERAPIST: Did you let your mom sit in the parking lot [at dance class]?

NATALIE: (*Looks down.*)

THERAPIST: What happened?

NATALIE: (*Looks down.*) I don't want to talk about it.

THERAPIST: Natalie, I like you just the same whether you have a good or bad week. If something is hard for you, we'll keep trying.

NATALIE: (*Looks up, sad expression.*) I cried. I wouldn't let her leave.

THERAPIST: It's okay. Did you let your mom hold her keys?

NATALIE: Yes, but I *held onto her.*

THERAPIST: You did try. That was more than you did last time. Natalie, if I told you a few weeks ago that soon you wouldn't need to call your mom or have her stay in school, what would you have said?

NATALIE: You're crazy (*giggles*).

THERAPIST: (*Smiles.*) Well, you did *let her go* . . . and *you can* let her leave dance class.

NATALIE: I can't. I don't want to come anymore. I already told my mom and dad.

THERAPIST: What did they say?

NATALIE: (*Sighs.*) I'm not coming.

THERAPIST: I don't expect you to *like* what we are doing. But you have to keep trying. So don't *tell me* that you don't need to come anymore—*show me*. When you can let your mom leave dance class . . . when you can take the school bus, go on play dates, and have a sleep-over, I'll be the first one to admit that we're done here.

NATALIE: (*Nods.*)

THERAPIST: Let's think about a better reward.

NATALIE: (*Smiles.*)

Overcoming Resistance

Use the Office

When working with youngsters with FAb/WCE, authentic exposures can be constructed in your office setting. For example, during sessions we might spontaneously ask youngsters to allow a parent to leave the waiting area and run an errand for a specified period of time. Typically, simply thinking or talking about such a scenario evokes a strong fear response. As a result, you can help youngsters negotiate their separation anxiety during in vivo exposures.

In our experience, most youngsters refuse to let a parent leave on the first attempt. In that case, the goals of the session are to facilitate a youngster's coping and to negotiate the details of the *next* session. Most youngsters, out of relief (of not being exposed), will surrender to some form of exposure during the next visit. Be sure to prepare parents for a youngster's resistance or even refusal to attend the next session.

Naturally, the degree of resistance will vary with each child. Some youngsters may allow a parent to run an errand as early as the second visit. (Of course, it helps if the errand involves picking up a small reward or tasty treat.) In Natalie's case, however, negotiating the office exposure was a slow, trying process. The sequence of exposures was as follows:

- Mrs. C. stays in the hallway (5 minutes).
- Mrs. C. steps outside the building; returns to hallway (10 minutes).
    Quick Check if needed.

- Mrs. C. takes a walk to nearby store; Natalie holds her keys (15 minutes).
- Mrs. C. takes a walk to a nearby store; keeps her keys (15–20 minutes).

During the last exposure, Natalie became hysterical. She refused to let her mother leave with her keys. "You'll get in the car and leave me!" she screamed. It was time to *change the dynamic*.

Change the Dynamic

For the next visit, we asked that Mr. C. bring Natalie to session. He did not tolerate her outbursts and was a weaker safety signal. As a result, Natalie allowed him to leave with his car for an unspecified amount of time.

Of course Natalie cried, but she stayed in the office and practiced her cognitive-based exercises. Some 30 minutes later, Mr. C. returned with a treat. Natalie remained calm the entire time. We praised her efforts and encouraged her to use this situation as *evidence* that her parents always return and that she could handle a spontaneous separation.

We successfully replicated the exposure during Natalie's dance class. The following session, we attempted the office exposure again with Mrs. C. This time, Natalie let her mother leave but insisted on holding the key to her house. We agreed, but Natalie understood that this was the *last time* she would be allowed such a safety signal.

Following the success of the office exposure, the next series of assignments involved play dates with familiar peers. Natalie had not been on a play date for months. As a result, to maintain her perception of control, the sequence of exposures was as follows:

- Mrs. C. stays for the entire time.
- Begin phase out: Mrs. C. stays for 30 minutes . . . 20 minutes . . . 10 minutes; promises to stay home.
- Mrs. C. leaves home; promises to stay local, and one phone call is allowed.
- Mrs. C. leaves home; vague as to whereabouts, and one phone call is allowed.
- Mrs. C. leaves home; vague as to whereabouts, and one emergency phone call is allowed.

Following the first few exposures, Natalie quickly progressed through the sequence. Given that she had had similar play dates in the past, she simply needed time to warm up to the routine.

Negotiating the Unfamiliar in the School Setting

"Get on the Bus"

Natalie did not take the school bus, nor did she carpool with family friends. Many parents such as Mrs. C. are willing to take their children to school as long as minimal disruption occurs. For others, however, taking youngsters to school is a major inconvenience and hassle.

We view taking the school bus as a *psychological* exposure similar to the basement exposure. Thus, not every youngster must take the bus. However, doing so, even periodically, is likely to enhance the child's perception of control. As you can imagine, Natalie became hysterical simply *thinking* about getting on the bus. Nevertheless, we wanted to help her ride the bus to enhance her school-related functioning, but also to prepare her for the inevitable daily bus ride of day camp in the next few months.

The first exposure was designed to maintain Natalie's perception of control; it consisted of the following:

- Mrs. C. helped Natalie get on the bus in the morning.
- Natalie sat toward the back of the bus and faced the rear window.
- Mrs. C. directly followed the bus in her car (visible to Natalie).
- Natalie took the bus home on her own.
- Mrs. C. promised to stay home during the day.

Natalie's first attempt was a success and did a great deal for enhancing her confidence. Thereafter, she was expected to take the bus to school on her own two times per week. In addition, Mrs. C. no longer promised to stay home. Rather, if pressed, she responded with "local" or "out of town." Following this sequence of exposures, carpooling to school with family friends was easily negotiated.

Negotiating the Unfamiliar in Other Settings

At this point, most youngsters are reasonably confident in their ability to negotiate separation-related scenarios. Unfamiliar play dates (i.e., new friend/house) and parties (new venues) can be set up in a similar fashion as the (vaguely) familiar play dates and dance exposure examples, respectively. As long as we maintained Natalie's perception of control, for example, she progressed through these exposures with minimal resistance. However, dealing with a new babysitter or a first-time sleep-over is likely to prove challenging.

The Babysitter

In our experience with separation-anxious youth, two common babysitter scenarios occur:

- Parents may limit socializing with friends; hence, a babysitter is rarely needed.
- Family has longstanding babysitter or close relative nearby.

The first scenario may stem from parental accommodation (i.e., gives in to youngster's fierce protests) or overprotection (i.e., fearful of leaving youngster with individuals other than family). In either case, the idea is to encourage parents to develop a more active social life (e.g., "you deserve it") and, at the same time, help their youngsters cope with FAb. The second scenario, although convenient, is too comfortable and may limit important opportunities for exposures.

The idea is not to displace loving relatives or close friends but to give them a *night off* and to create periodic challenges for youngsters. This can be accomplished by gradually introducing a new (trustworthy) babysitter. If at all possible, encourage parents to arrange brief babysitter visits (in their presence) with youngsters prior to the social engagement.

The next step could be short parental excursions (i.e., up to 1 hour) during the day or early evening, in which location, distance, and access to safety signals (e.g., super exposure) are all varied. This sets the stage for a full-fledged transitional exposure. Now parents can enjoy a regular night out without time constraints, and separation-anxious youngsters have their choice of safety signals. The process continues until youngsters are comfortable with a ration of one emergency phone call, which only the babysitter is allowed to make. Natalie was not thrilled with this process, but as long as we maintained her perception of control, she willingly attempted each exposure. Like the bus scenario, she found comfort in knowing that familiar babysitters (i.e., grandparents) would still be present *most of the time*.

"Please Don't Make Me Go"

For the separation-anxious youngster who worries about being abandoned, the grand finale exposure (due to the length of time the youngster is away from his or her parents) is the *sleep-over*. For this reason, we recommend the following sequence of exposures as a first step:

- Sleep-over at relative's house nearby (e.g., grandparent, aunt/ uncle)
- Sleep-over at relative's house farther away (i.e., within 1 hour)

Comment

These initial exposures serve as a transition to maintain a youngster's perception of control. Both scenarios may have occurred previously and involve a moderate sense of security. Nevertheless, given that resistance is likely, our goal is simply that the youngster willingly spends some minimal length of time (e.g., 1 hour) away from home at night. To accomplish this goal, the liberal use of safety signals (e.g., phone calls, parental promises to stay home, sibling accompanies the youngster) is acceptable. Be prepared for the possibility that youngsters may come home prematurely. This is more likely for youngsters with FAb/ FPI, who experience uncomfortable somatic complaints. For this reason, emphasize partial successes and a willingness to be exposed during child and parent sessions.

Once the family-related sleep-over is successfully negotiated, the more challenging peer-related sleep-over may be attempted. A good first choice is a close friend in the same neighborhood. Once again, provide safety signals as needed. The final exposure should be a sleepover at a friend's outside the neighborhood with minimal safety signals in place (i.e., one emergency phone call).

Natalie had minimal difficulty during the first sequence of exposures. Alternatively, she refused to sleep over at her best friend's house outside the neighborhood. She did, however, agree to a sleep-over at a later date. Of course, as that day approached, her separation anxiety became evident in her excuses to stay home.

To maintain Natalie's perception of control, we suggested that she go on an extended play date (i.e., stay for dinner) in which she could leave at any time. As the evening progressed, Natalie was asked if she'd like to sleep over. Mrs. C. encouraged her to stay over and offered an emergency phone call, if needed. In the end, Natalie slept over, had a great time, and did not return home until the following afternoon.

Negotiating the Unexpected

To truly minimize youngsters' FAb concerns, we must prepare them for, and help them to negotiate, unexpected separation-related scenarios. This approach is needed with any newly developed coping abilities.

In Natalie's case, Mrs. C. promised to pick her up after school on time or early. As long as Mrs. C. fulfilled her promise, Natalie did not experience any separation anxiety. But what if she were late?

In a previous example (see Dialogues 5.6 and 5.7), we helped Natalie examine the evidence *for* and *against* her mother's likelihood of being involved in a car accident. In Dialogue 10.3 we help Natalie explore alternative (healthy) explanations for those occasions when her mom is late and discuss problem-solving strategies.

Dialogue 10.3

Alternative explanations

THERAPIST: Natalie, what are some *good* reasons why your mom might pick you up late [from school]?

NATALIE: (*Shrugs shoulders.*)

THERAPIST: What kind of errands does your mom run?

NATALIE: She goes shopping.

THERAPIST: Could she get held up?

NATALIE: *Yes.* It's so slow [checking out]. I hate to go.

THERAPIST: What else could keep her from getting to you on time?

NATALIE: Traffic . . .

THERAPIST: Good. Anything else?

NATALIE: She's *always on the phone.*

THERAPIST: Could she lose track of time?

NATALIE: She does. I tell her to get off, but she yells at me for interrupting.

THERAPIST: (*Smiles.*) So, if your mom is late, does that mean she had a car accident?

NATALIE: (*Sighs, shakes head.*)

THERAPIST: What does it likely mean?

NATALIE: That she's shopping, stuck in traffic, or talking on the phone.

THERAPIST: Good.

Dysfunctional actions

THERAPIST: Natalie, what would you do if your mom was late?

NATALIE: (*Verge of tears*) I don't want her to be late.

THERAPIST: I'm not saying she will be late. But what would you do, if she were?

NATALIE: I'd run into the school building and call my mom's cell phone.

THERAPIST: What would you be doing?

NATALIE: I know (*sarcastic tone*), running away from my anxiety.

Alternative actions

THERAPIST: What could you do instead?

NATALIE: (*Shrugs shoulders.*)

THERAPIST: Could you *wait it out*?

NATALIE: For how long?

THERAPIST: Long enough to show yourself that your mom will come. This way, you *take away your anxiety* rather than waiting for your mom to take it away.

NATALIE: I guess I could wait a few seconds.

THERAPIST: *Natalie . . .*

NATALIE: A few minutes.

THERAPIST: That's better. And what should you do while you wait?

NATALIE: Talk to myself. Use my STOP.

THERAPIST: What would you say?

NATALIE: "*My mom always comes back.*"

THERAPIST: Good. What else could you do?

NATALIE: Wait with my best friend.

THERAPIST: How long should you wait before you call your mom?

NATALIE: Three minutes . . .

THERAPIST: *Natalie . . .*

NATALIE: Five minutes?

THERAPIST: That's good. But is 5 minutes really enough time if your mom gets stuck in line at the supermarket?

NATALIE: (*Shakes head.*)

THERAPIST: How about 10 minutes?

NATALIE: *Ten minutes . . .*

THERAPIST: I'm not saying that your mom will ever be 10 minutes late, but that's an appropriate amount of time to wait before thinking that something could be wrong.

NATALIE: Okay . . .

THERAPIST: So, if your mom is late, *what will you say to yourself?*

NATALIE: That she's shopping, stuck in traffic, or on the phone.

THERAPIST: And what will you do?

NATALIE: Wait 2 minutes (*giggles*) . . .

THERAPIST: *Natalie* . . .

NATALIE: Wait 10 minutes and stay with my friend.

THERAPIST: Great.

Parent Education

We prepared Mrs. C. to expect the following behaviors from Natalie as she began to *spontaneously* pick her up late from school:

- Hysterical outbursts
- Running into the school building
- Desperate demands to use the phone

To minimize Natalie's resistance, we set up the following sequence of exposures:

- Natalie is picked up *on time* the first 2 days.
- Natalie is picked up 1 minute late (Mrs. C. is present but out of view and can intervene, as necessary).
- Natalie is picked up early.
- Natalie is picked up on time.
- Natalie is picked up 2 minutes late (Mrs. C. is present but out of view).

During the next session, we emphasized partial successes and helped Natalie realize that she did *handle* her mother's lateness. The randomness of the exposures also modified Natalie's expectations that her mother would always be on time. We encouraged Mrs. C. to arrive late at least once per week to continue to enhance Natalie's perception of control.

The next step is to construct similar scenarios in other settings (e.g., play dates, parties). Prepare youngsters for the possibility of additional *late* outcomes. Use your judgment regarding the specific sequence of exposures needed. We recommend starting with a few familiar situations (i.e., play dates, extracurricular activities). At this point, Natalie experienced minimal separation anxiety as long as her mother showed up no more than 5 minutes late. Due to the randomness of the exposures, she came to realize that her mother's periodic lateness could be expected.

Comment

Natalie successfully negotiated both the *familiar* and *unfamiliar* scenarios in school and other settings. In addition, she was also equipped with the ability to handle unexpected outcomes. It was time to address termination issues, relapse prevention (discussed in Chapter 11), and the availability of future booster sessions. Four months later, Natalie had maintained her treatment gains. However, it was now the summer, and she was refusing to take the *camp* bus (but she was willing to attend camp).

Fear of Abandonment and Day Camp

Separation-related situations often emerge for youngsters attending day camp during the summer months. Referrals may come to your attention under the following circumstances:

- Sessions occur for the first time during the summer.
- Sessions overlap with the negotiation of school/other settings.
- Sessions occurred earlier in the year.

For our purposes, the second scenario is ideal. Negotiating camp-related situations builds on previous skills, further enhances a youngster's perception of control, and minimizes the likelihood of slips (see Chapter 11). The third scenario may stem from a resurgence of separation anxiety or a family's desire to reinforce the skills learned earlier in the year.

For illustrative purposes, however, we'll assume that you're meeting with the family for the first time. We'll also assume that youngsters will be attending camp for the first time or changing camps. Of course, any previous therapeutic contact or camp experience is likely to facilitate the outcome.

Making the Unfamiliar Familiar

As a general rule, youngsters with FAb/WCE are likely to become apprehensive *before* and *after* camp. For this reason, youngsters should:

- Spend time on the grounds before the start of camp.
- Visit (if possible) counselors/staff during the school year.
- Sign up with a friend.
- Engage in camp preparation activities (e.g., shopping for clothes/gear).

Although these activities will help prepare youngsters for the camp experience, at the same time, they are likely to trigger separation anxiety. Typically, youngsters with FAb/WCE prefer not to *think about* camp (i.e., being abandoned). Helping youngsters to focus on the more pleasant aspects of camp may minimize anticipatory abandonment fears.

Early preparation is also helpful for youngsters with FAb/FPI, who are likely to have more trouble *participating* in camp activities unless their safety signals are in place. Enhanced perception of control is likely to result from familiarization with the camp nurse, infirmary, office (with phone), counselors, dining hall, and location of bathrooms.

The Obligatory Camp Bus

Although taking the camp bus can be negotiated in a similar manner as our school-based example, the camp bus often proves more challenging for several reasons. For example, in our experience, most day camps discourage the practice of carpooling. Thus, we have less flexibility in modifying camp procedures to maintain a youngster's perception of control. In addition, given the obligatory nature of taking the camp bus, we cannot work with parents to plan (and control) exposures based on predictable arrival and departure times. As a result, youngsters may experience a diminished perception of control and heightened separation anxiety.

In Natalie's case, even though she had become accustomed to periodically taking the school bus, she became frantic simply thinking about the camp bus. Camp (and the bus) represented a novel and unfamiliar situation. To maintain Natalie's perception of control, we replicated the first school-based bus exposure. During the rest of the first week, Natalie willingly took the camp bus as long as Mrs. C. promised to stay home. During the second week, Mrs. C. no longer promised to stay home but responded to Natalie's questions about her proposed whereabouts with *local* or *out of town*. This approach did the trick until one chaotic afternoon when Natalie's bus arrived for departure 20 minutes late. She became hysterical and Mrs. C. was called to take her home. Natalie then refused to go back to camp.

Overcoming Resistance

During the next session, we validated Natalie's concerns, reframed the bus incident, and reviewed problem-solving strategies to prepare her for future late outcomes. With Mrs. C.'s support, we were firm about the need for Natalie to return to camp, but flexible regarding the temporary use of safety signals.

To minimize any further avoidance, Natalie was encouraged to return to camp over the weekend. The exposure consisted of having Natalie go swimming with her family as part of a weekend swim club. Mrs. C. was expected to run some spontaneous errands as Natalie remained with her father and brother. Most importantly, however, Mrs. C. was expected to be vague about her whereabouts and was expected to return late as well.

Another late but safe outcome in the camp context helped desensitize Natalie's fear of catastrophic consequences. When slips occur, the *timing* of subsequent exposures is crucial. If Natalie had been allowed to engage in avoidance, her separation anxiety would have become increasingly entrenched.

During the next week, Natalie willingly went to camp as long as she was allowed one emergency phone call. Thereafter, Natalie no longer mentioned a need for any safety signals.

Beware of Inclement Weather

In our experience, adverse weather conditions may exacerbate FAb-based separation anxiety. For example, thunder, lightning, and rain (and snow during the school year) may increase the likelihood of calamitous events. As a result, youngsters with WCE may refuse to attend camp (or school) to avoid worry about possible harm to caregivers (e.g., car accident). Alternatively, youngsters with FPI may refuse to take the camp (or school) bus due to an increased fear about their safety or increased likelihood of becoming physically ill (i.e., from motion sickness).

Natural environment-specific fears may serve as another manifestation of separation anxiety or may coexist as a full-fledged phobic disorder (Kendall et al., 2001). For the former, adverse weather conditions set the stage for *worst-case scenario* exposures and represent a form of overlearning for the separation-anxious youngster. During these circumstances, the initial liberal use of safety signals is recommended to encourage participation, which is then followed by their gradual elimination.

When separation anxiety coexists with a specific phobia, modifying the safety signals associated with abandonment fears is insufficient. For example, people with weather phobias (e.g., thunder/lightning, rain, snow) may experience a range of catastrophic cognitions (e.g., regarding the perceived imminence of flooding, fires, being struck by lightning) and avoidance behaviors (e.g., hide under bed, move to higher ground, excessive weather-channel viewing). As a result, *both* separation and weather-related fears need to be fully addressed either singly or in combination.

When Abandonment Fears Are Intense

For most youngsters, spending time away from home (e.g., summer camp) is a positive experience. Those with mild-to-moderate FAb may struggle with the bus or inclement weather during transitions. Others may experience mild homesickness (HS) (80–90%), which is considered a normal part of development (Thurber, Sigman, Weisz, & Schimdt, 1999). Severe HS (5–10%), however, is frequently associated with anxiety, depression, and social and behavioral problems (Thurber, 1995; Thurber et al., 1999). Youngsters may regularly stay in the camp office, cry, cling to counselors, and refuse to participate in activities.

Although the features of separation anxiety and HS may overlap (e.g., somatic complaints), HS can be distinguished from separation anxiety on several levels. For example, separation anxiety is primarily about the time preceding separation from people (e.g., caregivers, safe persons), whereas HS is primarily about the time following separation from home-related attachment persons and objects. In addition, separation anxiety typically involves anticipatory anxiety, whereas HS involves both anxiety and consequential depression (Thurber, 1995). In fact, youngsters with HS are more likely to experience elevated levels of negative emotion both prior to and subsequent to separations (Thurber et al., 1999).

For youngsters on the verge of attending day camp (with planned overnights) or sleepaway camp (to be discussed), features of both separation anxiety and HS should be integrated into the treatment process. Doing so will help foster coping skills, independence, and an increased sense of security with caregivers. Consider any of the following general recommendations to help facilitate a successful day-camp experience.

- Modify length of time/day in camp (morning, afternoon).
- Modify duration of camp session (2, 4, 6, or 8 weeks).
- Work with camp personnel (and parents) to facilitate transition and inclusion of safety signals.

In general, help parents and camp personnel to set realistic goals in light of separation anxiety and related problems. This way, despite separation anxiety, youngsters may still retain some degree of mastery.

FEARS OF BEING ALONE, OF ABANDONMENT, AND OF PHYSICAL ILLNESS

At intake, Felicia was terrified of vomiting and losing her breath. Her FPI largely maintained her fears of being alone and abandoned. She was reluctant to stay home alone or venture far from home because of the possibility of becoming physically ill. In addition, however, Felicia worried about the social consequences (e.g., embarrassment) of her fears. As a result, she received both relaxation and cognitive-based exercises. Given Felicia's behaviorally inhibited temperament and secure attachment, passive resistance and covert avoidance were expected.

Negotiating Staying Home Alone

For the most part, Felicia stayed home alone during the day. She quickly learned to adapt to the situation after school, since both parents worked. However, the television or radio served as a continuous distraction and created the illusion that she was not alone.

As a first step, we encouraged Felicia to spend an afternoon home alone without any electronic "crutches." She obliged, and for the first time, realized the extent of her separation anxiety. Unable to focus on her homework, she spent most of the afternoon talking with friends on the phone or surfing the Internet. In Dialogue 10.4 we discussed the importance of experiencing anxiety and the inhibiting effects of safety signals.

Dialogue 10.4

THERAPIST: Felicia, how was your afternoon [without electronic aids]?

FELICIA: (*Sighs.*) Terrible.

THERAPIST: How come?

FELICIA: I was so anxious. I used my inhaler *three* times.

THERAPIST: What did you think would happen?

FELICIA: I'd lose my breath.

THERAPIST: Did you have trouble catching your breath?

FELICIA: No.

THERAPIST: Have you used your inhaler before [when home alone in the afternoon]?

FELICIA: No . . .

THERAPIST: Why not?

FELICIA: I'm usually fine in the afternoon . . .

THERAPIST: As long as . . .

FELICIA: The TV or radio is on (*sighs*). Why do I *need to do that*?

THERAPIST: It's okay. It helps a lot of people to feel more secure. I'm not saying that you cannot listen to the TV or radio. However, I think it would be better if you used the exercises [breathing, relaxation, cognitive therapy] to *take away* your anxiety, and then listened to your programs. This way, *you* would be doing the coping.

FELICIA: (*Looks down.*)

THERAPIST: What's wrong?

FELICIA: I didn't exactly cope with my anxiety.

THERAPIST: What do you mean?

FELICIA: I was on the phone or the Internet until my mom came home.

THERAPIST: Again, that's okay. What I asked you to do wasn't easy. You were willing to try. Did you call your mom?

FELICIA: No, but I thought about it.

THERAPIST: You did great. Remember, it's a *good thing* for you to experience your anxiety. Try your best not to fight it. Should we try the assignment again?

FELICIA: (*Nods.*)

Comment

Felicia refrained from use of electronic aids upon arriving home from school during subsequent exposures. Each time she felt apprehensive, she was expected to wait 5 minutes (to experience the anxiety) before accessing a safety signal. During that time, we encouraged her to practice the exercises. To maintain her perception of control, Felicia was allowed to use her inhaler up to one time in the afternoon—unless, of course, she was having considerable difficulty breathing. In addition, she was allowed to use *one* electronic aid at a time to limit the degree of distraction (e.g., Internet, phone, radio, *or* television).

Worry about Calamitous Events versus Fear of Physical Injury

When staying home alone is primarily maintained by FPI (e.g., Felicia), treatment consists of the gradual removal of safety signals while preserving the adolescent's perception of control (i.e., minimal likelihood of physical illness). Given that an adolescent's home and surrounding accoutrements are potent safety signals, the therapeutic process is often met with passive forms of resistance.

Alternatively, when staying home alone is maintained by WCE, home-related safety signals have less value because the adolescent fears that his or her personal safety may be compromised (i.e., an intruder). In typical scenarios, an adolescent's resistance may be so strong that he or she has never been required to stay home alone. Imagine an older Michael at the time of intake. As a result, initial exposures may include any of the following:

- Parent takes a walk in the neighborhood (1–10 minutes).
- Parent visits a friend nearby (5–30 minutes).
- Parent runs an errand (5–30 minutes).

It is best to be prepared for a protracted and challenging experience, with many repeat exposures. Initially, the liberal use of safety signals is expected, especially access to a parent's cell phone. Unlike with youngsters who have FAb/WCE, being vague and spontaneous does little to heighten an adolescent's FBA-related separation anxiety. Rather, for youngsters with FBA (staying home alone)/WCE, the length of time alone and proximity of safety signals (e.g., takes parent longer to get home) assume critical importance. After all, the more time home alone, the greater the likelihood of a break-in.

As we moved through the FBA hierarchy, the real challenge was to convince Felicia's parents to go out more often. At night her parents regularly stayed home, even on the weekends. This was not a function of parental overprotectiveness but due to fatigue from the workweek and a desire to spend time as a family.

We encouraged Felicia's parents to go out socially at least one evening per week. They obliged and, in fact, soon looked forward to going out together and socializing with friends. Felicia expressed minimal resistance. Her parents became suspicious, however, when they noticed subtle changes to their bedroom upon arriving home (e.g., comforter slightly ruffled, magazines out of place, television left on a different channel). In Dialogue 10.5 we confronted Felicia regarding her *passive* (covert) avoidance behavior.

Dialogue 10.5

THERAPIST: How was the exposure [when parents went out to dinner] over the weekend?

FELICIA: (*Shrugs shoulders.*)

THERAPIST: Did you have trouble breathing?

FELICIA: Not really.

THERAPIST: Did you feel like you were going to throw up?

FELICIA: No.

THERAPIST: What did you do with yourself the entire time?

FELICIA: Hung out . . . called a friend.

THERAPIST: Did you call your parents?

FELICIA: No.

THERAPIST: Sounds like you did great?

FELICIA: (*Nods, smiles weakly.*)

THERAPIST: Where did you stay?

FELICIA: What do you mean?

THERAPIST: Which room in your house?

FELICIA: (*Looks down.*)

THERAPIST: Felicia . . .

FELICIA: (*Deep sigh*) My parents' bedroom.

THERAPIST: *Your parents' bedroom?* Why?

FELICIA: I don't know.

THERAPIST: Did it help you to feel safe?

FELICIA: (*Nods.*)

THERAPIST: It's okay. You *did* willingly let your parents go out, and they haven't done that for a while. But staying in their room was too comfortable. You didn't give yourself a chance to get anxious. What could you have done differently?

FELICIA: Stayed in my room and listened to the [relaxation] tape.

THERAPIST: That would have helped.

For the next exposure, we challenged Felicia's perception of control by encouraging her to stay in the finished attic. This room did not provide the same degree of comfort as her parents' bedroom, and even less than her own room. In addition, if loss of breath or physical illness emerged, she feared not being able to get help in time. We set up the exposure as follows:

- Wait 5 minutes before accessing a safety signal.
- Practice the diaphragmatic breathing (without tape).
- Listen to the relaxation tape, as needed.

To maintain her perception of control, she was allowed to use her inhaler one time unless her breathing became irregular. She was also allowed one emergency phone call.

Felicia successfully negotiated the attic exposure. She was able to regulate her breathing using the diaphragmatic exercises, but still chose to use her inhaler one time. We repeated the exposure (two more times) until Felicia could go without using her inhaler.

Negotiating her fear of staying home alone enhanced Felicia's confidence to tackle her abandonment fears. The crux of Felicia's separation anxiety stemmed from her FAb. Treatment sessions were structured in a similar manner as with Natalie.

Negotiating the Familiar in the School Setting

"Eat Your Breakfast"

To the casual observer, it did not appear that Felicia was experiencing school-related anxiety. However, she was neither eating nor drinking during breakfast or lunch in the school cafeteria. This abstinent behavior is common in children and adolescents who fear physical illness. The rationale, of course, is that it is less likely that the person will become ill with an empty stomach. Youngsters may feel insecure being away from home or parents and may not have access to suitable safe persons or signals. The problem, however, is that refusing to eat or drink is another form of avoidance and hence strengthens the separation anxiety.

Our first goal is to help youngsters eat or drink *something* for breakfast. The quantity is not important. Psychologically, anything that is consumed will heighten a youngster's FAb/FPI. Thus, you can maintain a youngster's perception of control (i.e., no pressure surrounding eating or drinking) by initially emphasizing some minimal limit, such as a half bowl of cereal or a half cup of milk. Some youngsters resist by drinking nothing but minimal quantities of water. This behavior represents a passive form of cheating (i.e., the youngster knows that he or she is less likely to become ill on water). For this reason, we find it is better to emphasize a more nutritive substance such as milk or juice.

Although Felicia was apprehensive about having breakfast, she willingly ate a half of a banana and drank a half cup of juice each morning. Within 3 days (without signs of physical illness), she was sufficiently confident to attempt eating in the cafeteria.

Comment

When youngsters refuse to eat or drink due to a fear of choking, similar procedures can be followed. Keep in mind, however, that choking is more likely than vomiting in the mind of a separation-anxious youngster. Any uncomfortable sensation in the throat may trigger FAb/FPI. As a result, you may need to proceed at a slower pace and pair relaxation/breathing procedures with each feeding opportunity. In addition, you may need to introduce or gradually eliminate a safe object (e.g., water bottle) to facilitate a youngster's coping.

The Cafeteria

When it comes to eating lunch in the school cafeteria, you may encounter any of the following circumstances:

- Refuses to eat.
- Goes home for lunch.
- Leaves campus for lunch (adolescents).
- Spends lunch period with school nurse (children).

We have two goals in mind. First, and most importantly, is to help youngsters gradually spend more time in the cafeteria. Keep in mind that simply being in the cafeteria often triggers unpleasant physical sensations. As a result, many youngsters will refuse to enter or stay in the cafeteria during lunch. This is especially true if strong social anxiety (i.e., embarrassing consequences of physical illness) accompanies the FAb/FPI. In some cases (e.g., older children and adolescents) it may be necessary to consider the following sequence of exposures:

- Enter and exit the cafeteria quickly during nonlunch hours (no one present).
- Observe cafeteria activity during lunch from entrance.
- Sit at lunch table with friends with no expectation to eat (does not bring lunch).

The second goal is for youngsters to eat or drink something in the cafeteria during lunch. Again, we emphasize partial successes to maintain a youngster's perception of control. Depending on the circumstances, it may not be necessary for a youngster to eat in the cafeteria *every* day. What's important, however, is that he or she is able do so. Each successful exposure weakens the association between unpleasant physical sensations and inevitable physical illness.

Felicia quickly felt comfortable eating breakfast each day as well as eating something in the cafeteria at least three times per week. Of course, it helped that several of her close friends (i.e., safe persons) sat at her table. In addition, she was careful to select easily digestible foods (e.g., fruit, yogurt). We challenged her perception of control when she ventured to restaurants (to be discussed).

Comment

When working with younger children (nursery/preschool to elementary), we recommend that they bring their lunch bag home at the end of the day. A youngster's idea of eating something (e.g., one unnoticeable bite of a sandwich) may differ from your own. In many cases, a youngster may eat nothing, throw out his or her lunch, and then distort his or her report of what was actually eaten. Although checking with a teacher or lunch monitor is often sufficient, viewing the remaining contents of a youngster's lunch bag helps hold him or her accountable.

The School Nurse

Children (again, nursery/preschool to elementary) with FAb/FPI may spend an inordinate amount of time in the nurse's office. For example, they may visit during morning transitions (i.e., drop-off times), performance-oriented situations (e.g., tests, gym) or unstructured times (lunch, recess) when physical sensations are likely to be triggered. Because the school nurse may play a pivotal role in helping youngsters to overcome their separation anxiety, it may be important to familiarize him or her or the school with a youngster's arsenal of coping strategies. For example, a copy of the relaxation tape and some STOP stickers could be made available so that the nurse could help facilitate the child's coping. We also recommend that the school nurse consider any of the following strategies:

- Using the VRI acronym to shape youngster's behavior (practice coping strategies).
- Requiring clear indices of physical illness (i.e., elevated thermometer reading) to remain in the nurse's office.

- Making time spent in the office unattractive (e.g., planned ignoring).
- Having the youngster spend time with less familiar school personnel (e.g., principal).
- Employing a school-based reward system for spending less time in nurse's office.

In some cases, however, youngsters may cling to a safe object (e.g., water bottle) or place (e.g., bathroom) to avoid his or her anxiety, rather than visit with the school nurse.

The Bathroom

For youngsters with FAb/FPI, the bathroom (i.e., school and other public settings) can be a potent safety signal. For example, some youngsters simply need to know where the bathrooms are at all times, just in case they became physically ill. This preference tends to be more characteristic of older children and adolescents who for social (anxiety) reasons would rather not visit the nurse. Felicia always made sure she was in close proximity to a bathroom.

In other cases, some youngsters' FPI may be manifested in the fear of losing bladder control. The slightest sensation may prompt excessive bathroom use, and youngsters may stay nearby safe persons or bathrooms to minimize the possibility of having an accident. In either situation, our goal is to gradually replace safe persons, objects, and places with prescriptive coping skills.

Negotiating the Familiar in Other Settings

As we moved through the hierarchy, we helped Felicia negotiate familiar situations such as eating in restaurants, going to the movies, and taking car trips. Like Natalie, these situations were familiar, though *vaguely*, because Felicia rarely participated. Due to her FAb/FPI, Felicia did not express interest in these activities. Of course, it didn't help matters that her parents were content to stay at home.

During the first exposure, Felicia went to the local diner. To maintain her perception of control, we agreed to the following conditions:

- Go with parents.
- Does not have to eat or drink.
- Can take bronchial inhaler.
- Can sit at table near the restrooms.

After being seated, Felicia's parents reported that she looked flushed, refrained from conversation, kept her hand in her pocket (i.e., holding inhaler), and watched the restrooms. This lasted about 20 minutes, when her parents' food arrived. Shortly thereafter, Felicia struggled to breathe, stood up, then demanded to leave. Her parents tried to calm her, but Felicia bolted for the door.

Overcoming Resistance

Get Back on the Horse

Problematic exposures can be highly therapeutic as long as they are reframed properly and occur in the context of the treatment program. In Dialogue 10.6, we helped Felicia evaluate the diner exposure in a *healthy* way.

Dialogue 10.6

THERAPIST: Felicia, how did the [diner] exposure go?

FELICIA: (*Sighs, purses her lips.*) Terrible . . . I hate feeling like this. Why should I even bother anymore?

THERAPIST: I know it's difficult . . . but you *did* go to the diner. How long did you stay?

FELICIA: Twenty minutes.

THERAPIST: That's great! When was the last time you went to the diner?

FELICIA: It's been a while . . .

THERAPIST: In all honesty, you did better than I anticipated.

FELICIA: (*Weak smile*) *Really?*

THERAPIST: That's right. We didn't set a time limit. You *willingly* went to the diner and stayed for *20 minutes.* That's a long time for someone who fears physical illness. Did you use your inhaler?

FELICIA: No, but I held onto it in my pocket.

THERAPIST: That's okay. Did you go to the bathroom?

FELICIA: No, but I thought about it.

THERAPIST: You really challenged yourself this time.

FELICIA: *I did?*

THERAPIST: That's right. You're too hard on yourself.

FELICIA: (*Sighs.*) I know . . .

THERAPIST: The key is not to fight your anxiety but to expect it and be prepared for it.

FELICIA: (*Nods.*)

THERAPIST: What happens when you fall off a horse?

FELICIA: You get back on . . .

THERAPIST: You bet. Did you think by now that you would be eating breakfast and having lunch in the cafeteria?

FELICIA: (*Shakes head.*)

THERAPIST: Remember, there is nothing that you cannot do. You just *think* that way. And that's your anxiety. What will you do next time?

FELICIA: Stay longer.

THERAPIST: You don't have to stay longer. The key is not to leave at the *height of your anxiety*. How can you help yourself?

FELICIA: Practice my breathing. Talk to myself.

THERAPIST: If necessary, you can go to the bathroom, even take a walk outside to get some air. At the very least, try to stay on the grounds of the diner until you feel calm. This way, you will habituate to your anxiety. During the next exposure your anxiety will begin at a lower level. Are you ready to try again?

FELICIA: (*Nods.*)

THERAPIST: I didn't hear you.

FELICIA: Yes (*tries to hold back smile*).

Parent Education

For the next exposure, we encouraged Felicia's parents to help their daughter remain at the diner until she was calm. Once again, Felicia was not expected to eat anything, and her safety signals were in place to maintain her perception of control. As a transition, we suggested that Felicia bring along a comfort food of her own (e.g., yogurt). We conveyed that it was completely up to her if she wanted to attempt to eat something.

Surprisingly, Felicia stayed at the diner for over an hour, ate her yogurt, and even sampled some of her mother's soup. Her parents reported that, at times, that Felicia practiced her breathing exercises, got up and walked around, and vigilantly watched the bathroom. Overall, she appeared most pleased with her accomplishment.

During the next series of exposures, we modified Felicia's safety signals and the persons present. For example, she went back to the diner and another familiar restaurant (but farther away from home) with different friends and their families. She also sat farther away from the restrooms. She was expected to order and eat her own meals. We allowed her one emergency phone call to her parents, if needed.

Felicia successfully negotiated each of the exposures. She was now ready to attempt unfamiliar restaurants (to be discussed) and familiar (but often avoided) car trips.

Car Trips

For youngsters with FAb/FPI, car trips can be considered ultimate exposures for several reasons. First, any form of FPI (vomiting, choking, bathroom-related accidents) can be addressed. Second, car trips can easily heighten FPI in the following ways:

- Deny access to safe persons, signals, or places.
- Increase likelihood of motion sickness.
- Diminish perception of control as a passenger.

Third, the therapist can intensify the FAb by modifying any of the safety signals. Most youngsters with FAb/FPI avoid car trips of 30 minutes or longer. This was certainly true of Felicia. For this reason, the first sequence of *familiar* exposures involved Felicia's parents and consisted of the following:

- Driving around town (local) for 30 minutes.
- Driving to a (familiar) mall 1 hour away.
- Taking a family trip to visit relatives 3 hours away.

As you can imagine, the third exposure would likely give Felicia the most difficult time, even in the presence of her parents. She willingly participated but at times begged her parents to pull over because she was feeling sick. To help maintain her perception of control, her parents were allowed to do so one time. On the way home, however, they agreed to drive straight through; Felicia successfully negotiated this sequence of exposures.

The second sequence of exposures involved driving to familiar places (i.e., at least 1 hour away) with *safe* friends and their families. Naturally, pulling over was not acceptable for social (anxiety) reasons. Felicia used her inhaler one time during the first car trip but successfully used her breathing exercises during the second trip. She was now ready to take on more challenging *unfamiliar* exposures.

Comment

When FAb is maintained by a fear of having a bathroom-related accident, consider having youngsters drink frequently during car trips. This will show youngsters that they're unlikely to have an accident even during the most probable circumstances. As a result, the FAb/FPI will likely diminish considerably.

In addition, if relevant, consider having youngsters attend movies of different durations without allowing bathroom access. Once again, eating or drinking during these engagements serve our purposes. As with car trips, start with family members as companions and then lessen the degree of familiarity.

Negotiating the Unfamiliar in the School Setting

School-Related Sporting Events (Spectator)

Although Felicia was athletic and an avid member of her school's track team, she rarely attended school-related sporting events. Her FPI and social anxiety kept her close to home or her parents and was adversely affecting her friendships. With some encouragement, Felicia was now willing to attend school-related sporting events. To maintain her perception of control, we set up the following sequence of exposures:

- Attend with best friend (at her school for 30, 60, and 90 minutes).
- Attend with best friend (at other familiar schools for 60 and 90 minutes).
- Attend with good friend and eat/drink something (no time limit).
- Attend by self (at her school for 30 minutes).
- Attend by self and eat/drink something (at her school for 60 minutes).

After the success of the car-trip exposures, Felicia had minimal difficulty until the third exposure. As a result of her heightened anxiety, she was allowed to choose her safety signals. For example, rather than purchase unfamiliar foods from a vendor, she brought her own. In addition, she also requested that her parents remain home just in case she became physically ill.

The last two exposures were challenging, but Felicia negotiated them as long as her perception of control was maintained. For example, during the fourth exposure, Felicia insisted that one of her parents remain in the parking lot as she attended the sporting event. We agreed as long as she was willing to attempt the last exposure with minimal safety signals in place.

During the final exposure, Felicia was expected to attend a sporting event at her school alone (60 minutes) and eat vendor-purchased food. In addition, her parents were not required to stay home. Felicia's sole safety signal would be one emergency phone call (if needed) to her parents.

Much to our amazement, Felicia stayed for the entire event (2 hours), ate some french fries, and did not need to call her parents. It turned out, unexpectedly, that one of her friends from another school attended as well; Felicia reported feeling like she had cheated during the exposure (i.e., she had spent time with her friend). We praised Felicia's efforts and honesty (i.e., no more passive resistance) and gave her complete credit for the exposure. After all, she had no way of knowing the composition of the attendees. She was now ready to negotiate similar scenarios but with *unfamiliar* elements or settings.

Negotiating the Unfamiliar in Other Settings

During this part of the program, we set up unfamiliar exposures by modifying the safety signals and emphasizing the venues of restaurants and car trips.

Restaurants

Felicia attended novel restaurants (local and out of town) and digested foods that she perceived more likely to induce physical illness (e.g., fish, tacos). Naturally, to maintain her perception of control and to further enhance her confidence, the first few exposures involved her parents. Thereafter, she ventured to unfamiliar eateries with persons who varied in their degree of perceived support. Felicia experienced minimal difficulty during these exposures and actually enjoyed trying new foods. She was astonished as to how far she had come since the initial diner exposure.

Getting Lost on a Car Trip

Regarding car trips, we varied the distance, location (i.e., small villages to completely rural areas), and persons involved. Once again, we started with Felicia's parents. When it came time to take a drive *in the middle of nowhere*, we encouraged Felicia's parents to act as if they were lost for a brief interval (i.e., 1 minute). Use your judgment when attempting this tactic. Keep in mind that being lost may greatly diminish a separation-anxious youngster's perceived control. For most youngsters, simply being in a rural area is a sufficient exposure. Given Felicia's progress, we felt such a challenge, if properly executed, would further enhance her perception of control.

Initially, as expected, Felicia started to panic. However, with some assistance from her mother and by using the exercises, she was able to regulate her breathing. In session, we reframed the situation as a *worst-case scenario*, in which she successfully coped without using her inhaler.

After Felicia processed what had happened, she expressed minimal fear regarding forthcoming car trips. This turned out to be true as she effortlessly completed the next series of exposures with persons other than her parents. Of course, this set the stage for the next challenge.

Professional Sports Event

As much as Felicia enjoyed watching professional sports on television, she had never actually attended a live sporting event. The prospect of venturing far from home (with or without her parents) to a completely unfamiliar place with massive numbers of fans hardly appealed to her.

Surprisingly, out of the blue, one of her relatively close friends invited her to attend a much sought-after event in another city. Naturally, Felicia was ambivalent. However, with some encouragement and the support of her parents, she accepted the invitation.

At this point, Felicia was relatively convinced that she would not become physically ill, nor would she need to use her inhaler. Nevertheless, given the magnitude of the exposure, Felicia took her inhaler as well as her parents' cell phone.

Felicia was thrilled to report that she had had a wonderful time at the sporting event. She also reported that she had not needed to use the cell phone or the inhaler. Indeed, this accomplishment was quite remarkable considering that she was sitting in a "nose bleed" section of the arena. Felicia expressed excitement about the possibility of attending another sports event in the near future. She appeared ready to contemplate the ultimate unfamiliar FAb event: attending sleepaway camp.

Fear of Abandonment and Sleepaway Camp

When it comes to attending sleepaway camp, we typically encounter two scenarios involving separation-anxious youth:

- Previously experienced unsuccessful camp experience (i.e., came home prematurely).
- Never attended sleepaway camp.

Both scenarios can be handled similarly because youngsters in either category are likely to express minimal or no desire to attend. For the first scenario, however, you are more likely to have the support of parents. For the second scenario, although it may be therapeutic for separation-anxious youth to attempt attending sleepaway camp, ambivalence about the undertaking is typical between spouses (i.e., indulgent versus controlling). Use your judgment to determine whether attending sleepaway camp should be part of the program. For now, let's address the circumstances of a previously unsuccessful camp experience.

If we left it up to the youngster, the word *camp* would never be mentioned again. So why bother? We believe that youngsters need a *corrective* experience; otherwise, forthcoming extended separations (from parents or home) may also be dreaded, and adjustment is likely to be poor.

As a first step, it's important to help youngsters reframe the first camp experience in a healthy way that emphasizes effort and partial successes. Simply attending camp for the first time, for any length of time, is commendable. Perhaps any of the following variables adversely affected a youngster's experience:

- Age (too young)
- Poor fit (interests, activities, peers, counselors)
- Lack of perceived support (from home and at camp)
- Distance from home
- Separation anxiety, homesickness, and related problems

We focus on how the next camp experience is likely to be better in terms of the camp itself as well as the youngster's newly developed coping skills.

Felicia's first sleepaway camp experience occurred 3 years ago. The camp was 5 hours away and she went without the benefit of having a friend attend with her. Although slated to attend for 4 weeks, her separation and social anxieties as well as homesickness got the best of her. After 3 short days, she came home with an attitude to never return.

As you can imagine, Felicia was not too keen about the idea of trying sleepaway camp again. In our view, it wasn't crucial that she actually attend, only that she *think* she might. For example, we encouraged her to conduct Internet-based camp searches as well as having camp-related discussions both in session and at home. Such tactics discourage youngsters from engaging in mental blocking.

Because our goal is to facilitate a corrective experience, neither the length of time nor the distance from home is crucial. Sleepaway camp experiences of 1 week are sufficient. In addition, if it helps, look for camps located within a 1-hour radius of the youngster's home.

Despite finding a 1-week program that was within 30 minutes, Felicia was still hesitant. The clincher came when one of her friends decided to attend the camp as well. With the support of her parents, we helped Felicia willingly (and officially) sign up for camp. Typically, the process leading up to sending in the deposit is often more therapeutic than the actual camp experience.

At this point, the process of termination could ordinarily have begun, given Felicia's progress and the fact that sleepaway camp was several months away. However, we still needed to address her interoceptive avoidance more fully.

Negotiating Interoceptive Avoidance

Although Felicia was not avoiding running track, she was *holding back* due to fear of hyperventilation. Previous exposures (e.g., being alone, eating in restaurants, taking car trips) were associated with interoceptive avoidance. However, there was never any *real* threat that Felicia would hyperventilate or vomit.

Regarding track, however, the act of physical exertion made her feared sensations all the more plausible. As a result, we needed to expose her to situations that would diminish her sensitivity to these feared physical sensations. This could be accomplished in much the same way as individuals with panic disorder undergo symptom-induction tests (see Barlow, 2002).

As a first step, we chose tests that mimicked a loss of breath or hyperventilation in the office. These included running in place (2 minutes), stair stepping (1 minute), and breathing through a thin straw (2 minutes). Our purposes were twofold: (1) to show Felicia that physical exertion would not lead to hyperventilation, and (2) to help Felicia use the breathing/relaxation exercises to restore her perception of control rather than the use of her inhaler. Upon the successful completion of these procedures, Felicia was ready to exert herself at home (e.g., treadmill), the gym, track practice, and track meets.

Naturally, we were careful to maintain her perception of control. We gradually modified her safety signals by varying the degree of physical exertion, proximity of safe persons or settings, and the use of her inhaler.

As a first step, Felicia gradually increased the speed/degree of incline on her treadmill at home. She willingly refrained from the use of her inhaler as long as a parent was in the house. This progress led to gym workouts (with a personal trainer) and track practice (at three-quarters exertion) without using her inhaler. This was a major step: Previously, Felicia had *always* used her inhaler prior to practice, irrespective of the need to do so.

As we moved through the hierarchy, Felicia challenged herself while running in the neighborhood. During the first exposure, her mother followed her in the car. For the second exposure, Felicia braved the roads alone as long as her mother stayed home and Felicia had both inhaler and cell phone in her pocket.

Overcoming Resistance

The big test came during her first track meet. Felicia willingly refrained from using her inhaler prior to the race. Unfortunately, she held back considerably and came in last place. Distraught and out of breath, Felicia quit the track team. In Dialogue 10.7, we helped her reevaluate the outcome.

Dialogue 10.7

FELICIA: I quit the track team.

THERAPIST: Why? You were doing great.

FELICIA: I came in last place (*deep sigh*).

THERAPIST: Did you use your inhaler?

FELICIA: No, but what difference does it make?

THERAPIST: What have we been working on?

FELICIA: Not being afraid to run without my inhaler.

THERAPIST: That's right. Have you been using your inhaler?

FELICIA: No.

THERAPIST: Are you still afraid?

FELICIA: Not really.

THERAPIST: That's not remarkable?

FELICIA: I guess so, but I came in last.

THERAPIST: I know that's disappointing. But was it reasonable to think you wouldn't hold back at all during your first race?

FELICIA: No.

THERAPIST: What are we emphasizing here?

FELICIA: My willingness to try.

THERAPIST: That's right. As far as I'm concerned, you won the race.

FELICIA: (*Weak smile*)

THERAPIST: Why do you run track?

FELICIA: To stay in shape and be with my friends.

THERAPIST: Has that changed?

FELICIA: No.

THERAPIST: Do you want to give that up?

FELICIA: Not really.

THERAPIST: Are you worried about what others may think?

FELICIA: (*Nods.*)

THERAPIST: Is there any evidence that people are talking about you?

FELICIA: If anything, they are very supportive. (*Sighs.*)

THERAPIST: What's wrong?

FELICIA: Nothing. I'm not fast.

THERAPIST: You don't have to be. Remember, you're your own baseline. Keep working hard and set your own goals. Do you need to talk to the coach?

FELICIA: No.

THERAPIST: You don't want to stay on the team?

FELICIA: I do. I never told him I quit.

THERAPIST: (*Smiles.*)

Fear of Abandonment and Fear of Physical Injury: The Path to Panic and Agorophobia?

It certainly looked as if Felicia were moving toward developing panic disorder and agoraphobia. For example, prior to treatment she experienced a broad range of agoraphobic avoidance (e.g., regarding being alone, taking car trips, eating in restaurants, attending sports events).

In addition, she also clung tightly to safe persons, places, situations, and objects.

She was not yet quite in the realm of panic disorder in the sense that her interoceptive avoidance was limited (i.e., to vomiting and hyperventilation), her panic-like reactions were cued (expected), and her panic-related cognitions were not fully developed. Nevertheless, the potential for developing uncued full-spectrum panic attacks was there. For example, during an unplanned follow-up visit, Felicia reported her first *unexpected*, limited-symptom panic attack. In Part VI we help youngsters and their families stay in control despite pitfalls and relapse.

PART VI

NAVIGATING THE OBSTACLE COURSE

In Chapter 11 we present guidelines for helping children and their families stay in control despite pitfalls (comorbidity and treatment implementation issues) and relapse. In addition, we consider the merits of pharmacotherapy, address termination issues, and introduce relapse prevention exercises to facilitate generalization and maintenance of treatment outcomes.

CHAPTER II

Staying in Control

Managing Pitfalls and Relapse

Why does this keep happening to me? I'll never be normal. (*Sighs*.)
—FELICIA

THE CHALLENGE OF COMORBIDITY

The majority of youngsters with separation anxiety experience mild-to-moderate comorbid problems. This was true for Brian (OCD symptoms), Felicia (social anxiety), Michael (generalized anxiety), and Natalie (generalized anxiety). When severe problems co-occur, however, a short-term coping-oriented anxiety-management program may be insufficient (Eisen & Silverman, 1998; Kendall et al., 2001; Southam-Gerow, Weisz, & Kendall, 2003). Under these circumstances, more comprehensive programs are needed that address both separation anxiety and related problems.

We have found that OCD and learning disorders frequently co-occur with separation anxiety, and if severe, may significantly disrupt treatment outcome. In this section, we discuss both problems and provide suggestions for modifying your treatment program. Let's begin with a discussion of OCD.

Obsessive–Compulsive Disorder

It's not surprising that OCD-related symptoms often co-occur with separation anxiety. Youngsters with both separation anxiety and OCD may fear being alone or abandoned due to preoccupation with images of harm to themselves or others (Geller et al., 1996). The worry/obsessive thought content of OCD is, by nature, intrusive (e.g., morbid imagery of violence and death), pervasive, and triggered by a range of superstitious events. Separation-related worries, however, are typically less intricate (e.g., car accident, break-in) and occur in anticipation of separation from caregivers.

OCD is also associated with compulsive behaviors (e.g., washing hands, checking doors, locks, or whatever is the focus), whereas separation anxiety is associated with safety signals. Naturally, the two may overlap. For example, when safety signals are not present (e.g., alone in the basement), the youngster may develop rituals as an alternative way of reducing his or her anxiety. This was the case for Brian. However, when the ritualistic activity becomes time consuming (i.e., more than 1 hour per day), consider any of these courses of action.

- Negotiate separation anxiety as a first step.
- Negotiate OCD along the way (build momentum).
- Negotiate separation anxiety and OCD concurrently.

Within this framework, our approach to managing compulsions is three-pronged. First, we encourage youngsters to *wait out the urge*, that is, to spend increasing amounts of time waiting to perform the (complete) ritual. At this point, the youngster may experience anxiety but his or her perception of control is maintained because the ritual *can* still be performed. The longer the wait, the weaker the urge or need to perform the ritual. As long as you do not place a restriction on the number of rituals to be performed, youngsters may wait for extended intervals (an hour) before performing rituals. With enough waiting intervals spread throughout the day, the number of rituals is reduced indirectly. This reduction sets the stage for helping youngsters to *knowingly* cut back the specific number of rituals they perform per day.

As a second step, consider interrupting rituals to avoid closure (e.g., wash one hand). Once again, to maintain a youngster's perception of control, emphasize a general time frame. Initially, the youngster can still complete the ritual. Once his or her urges weaken through waiting, you can reduce the number of completed rituals to be performed.

The third and most important step is to help youngsters cut back rituals by emphasizing a specific number to be performed (e.g., skip ritual every other time). Be sure to focus on partial successes and replace safety signals or rituals with any of the cognitive-behavioral therapy exercises discussed thus far. Consider using rewards when ritual reduction proves difficult (e.g., obsessive focus on mental rituals such as rationalizing or praying) or a youngster's resistance is strong (see Fitzgibbons & Pedrick, 2003; for specific guidelines when OCD is the primary disorder, see March & Mulle 1998).

Learning Disorders

Learning disorders (LDs) can also have far reaching effects in academic, social, and behavioral domains (e.g., Sorenson et al., 2003). Deficits may occur in visual perception, speech/language, verbal and nonverbal memory, planning, and motor development. Approximately one-third of youngsters who have LDs may experience internalizing problems (Greenham, 1999). If youngsters appear to have difficulty attending to or retaining treatment-session content, they may have weaknesses in the following areas:

- Central/auditory processing
- Short-term memory
- Limited abstract thinking abilities

Youngsters may have difficulty understanding treatment goals and homework assignments when processing or memory-related deficits are operating. This hitch may be especially likely when it comes to receiving contingent rewards (e.g., "You didn't say that"). Misinterpretations may cause youngsters undue frustration. It doesn't help matters when a parent perceives his or her youngster as difficult, manipulative, and spoiled. In essence, however, the youngster may have processed the deal differently and truly believes that his or her view is correct. Consider the following suggestions to help youngsters get the most out of your treatment sessions.

- Use clear and simple language and break down exercises into small steps.
- Provide frequent clarifications regarding session content, exercises, goals, and rewards (e.g., "What is your homework assignment again?").
- Provide frequent repetition and practice of cognitive-behavioral therapy strategies.

- Ask questions to ensure understanding ("What does the STOP sign stand for again?").
- Rely on contingency contracts to avoid misinterpretations.
- Present session material using a variety of sensory modalities (auditory, visual, kinesthetic).

In addition to attending to sessions and retaining treatment-session content, we have found that youngsters with learning issues may also have limited abstract thinking abilities. If this limitation is evident, it will be important to make session content as concrete as possible. For example, regardless of a youngster's age, consider using easels and cartoon strips to illustrate session content (Kendall, 1990).

Exposure-based homework assignments should also be as specific as possible (e.g., time, place, duration, expected outcome). Imaginal exposures are likely to be too abstract. To avoid confusion and undue frustration on the family's part, consider simulating exposures in session. For example, our *office exposure* (see Chapter 10) is quite authentic and helps give youngsters a clear idea of what to expect during the week; hence, they may experience a heightened perception of control and a greater likelihood of successful coping.

In our work with anxious youth, we see a disproportionate number of youngsters with nonverbal learning disorders (NLD). Youngsters with NLD are twice as likely to be diagnosed with an internalizing disorder than youngsters with verbal learning disorders (Petti, Voelker, Shore, & Hayman-Abello, 2003). Ten percent of the LD population has NLD (Rourke, 1995).

NLD is often identified by a verbal-performance split of at least 20 points on a standardized IQ test and is associated with weaknesses in visual attention and perception, physical coordination, adaptability, organizational skills, mental flexibility (i.e., dichotomized thinking), and nonverbal communication (i.e., interpreting social cues; Stewart, 2002; for a full explication regarding diagnosis and treatment, see Tanguay, 2001).

Given this profile, it's not surprising that NLD frequently co-occurs with OCD or SAD. Regarding OCD, there may be a subtle neurocognitive basis for weaker nonverbal reasoning skills (Cox, Fedio, & Rapoport, 1989). Behaviorally, however, the often confusing and unpredictable world associated with NLD sets the stage for clinging to rituals or safety signals to restore some sense of personal control. If you suspect learning or attentional issues, consider a psychoeducational assessment to determine the nature of the deficits and whether a Section 504 (i.e., individualized educational plan [IEP] is warranted in the school setting.

Overall, it's important to remember that youngsters with separation anxiety may also experience:

- Comorbid internalizing and externalizing problems
- Learning or attentional issues
- Insecure-ambivalent attachment
- Behavioral inhibition
- Low frustration tolerance

Because of this comorbid complexity, we find it helpful to design structured and concrete programs that afford flexibility and maintain youngsters' perception of control. Regardless of the circumstances, it is best to start with the familiar and predictable, then gradually move toward the unfamiliar and the unexpected. By doing so, you will facilitate youngsters' adaptability as well as helping them negotiate separation anxiety and related problems.

Although comorbidity can be a major obstacle in thwarting positive outcome, treatment implementation issues can also lead you off course. In the next section, we discuss child and parent factors that may affect motivation for, and compliance with, the treatment program.

TREATMENT IMPLEMENTATION ISSUES

Lack of Motivation

Separation-anxious youth often lack motivation to participate in a treatment program. This is not surprising given that we are asking them to *give up* their security for the promise of learning prescriptive coping skills. For example, younger children may not understand why they cannot continue to sleep in the parental bed. This is especially true if parental accommodation has been long-standing. Youngsters may go along with initial exposures as long as their perception of control is maintained and a prized reward is part of the deal. However, once the exposures become truly anxiety provoking, rewards may lose their value and resistance may become fierce. Creative strategies (e.g., walkie-talkie, baby monitor) to help maintain youngsters' perception of control are useful as they work their way through the exposures. In addition, therapeutic goals should be discussed in the context of greater responsibilities and independence as they become older. Rewards should also emphasize the privileges associated with greater maturity.

Older children and adolescents are more likely to understand the goals of the treatment program. However, *accepting* and making a *com-*

mitment toward these goals is another story, especially if they are strong-willed or possess a behaviorally inhibited temperament (i.e., more likely to cheat during exposures). Your coach persona will help build youngsters' confidence, hold them accountable for their actions, and minimize aversive parent–child power struggles.

Noncompliance

A youngster's motivation naturally improves as each step of the treatment program is successfully carried out. Persistent noncompliance, however, can easily thwart treatment progress.

Youngsters are more likely to be noncompliant if they view the exposures as too anxiety provoking. Remember, all-or-nothing thinking (see Chapter 5) is frequently characteristic of separation-anxious youth. When these youngsters cannot visualize coping with an exposure, they are likely to shut down and refuse to make an effort. This unwanted possibility is why maintaining a youngster's perception of control is so important. Exposures should be framed in terms of partial successes and willingness to participate.

Noncompliance may also stem from a youngster's view that treatment sessions or procedures are too unpleasant or a nuisance. For these reasons, consider making the components of the treatment program as attractive as possible through the application of contingent reinforcers (see Chapter 7) and the therapeutic use of game play (see Kaduson & Schaefer, 1997, 2001).

Naturally, parental noncompliance is of greater concern; if severe, it can be responsible for treatment failure. If any of the following occur, you may need to reevaluate a family's commitment to the treatment program (Eisen & Kearney, 1995).

- Repeated cancellations of intake or treatment sessions
- Refusal to complete questionnaires/handouts
- Failure to follow through with exposure-based homework assignments
- Failure to properly dispense contingent rewards

Typically, however, parental noncompliance is less direct and explicit; instead it is reflected in a parent's nominal efforts—he or she merely *goes through the motions* of the treatment procedures. This subtler form of noncompliance may stem from overprotectiveness, a high-intensity temperament, or unrealistic expectancies regarding treatment outcome.

For example, some parents (e.g., Michael's mother) may have difficulty understanding or accepting our rationale for placing youngsters in separation anxiety-provoking scenarios. Our view that youngsters need to become *more anxious* initially may be received as disheartening news. In some instances, a parent may be unable to tolerate the youngster's distress. As a result, he or she may continue to give both verbal and nonverbal reassurances during exposures, making habituation to separation anxiety less likely to occur. In this case, special attention should be devoted to educating and helping parents reduce their accommodations during exposures. In addition, the sequence of exposures may need to be more gradual in nature, so that both child *and* parent can handle the degree of distress. Finally, if at all possible, utilize others who can adopt calm postures during the exposures.

Noncompliance may also be the result of a parent's own high-intensity temperament (e.g., Natalie's mother). A parent with low frustration tolerance, a competitive nature, and a serious disposition may easily become disenchanted with his or her youngster's lack of progress. To complicate matters, escalating power struggles are likely to ensue when a youngster possesses a similar (strong-willed) temperamental style.

If you suspect that a parent's high-intensity temperament is negatively impacting treatment outcome, consider administering our Playfulness Scale for Adults (PSA; Schaefer & Greenberg, 1997; see Appendix I). Sample items include "I consider myself to be a serious, no-nonsense type of person" (reverse scoring) and "I like to smile and laugh as much as possible during the day."

To enhance parental playfulness, consider concurrently assigning weekly family game-playing (noncompetitive) activities. Doing so will likely help parents relate more effectively and patiently to their youngsters and enhance cooperative treatment efforts.

Sometimes noncompliance may result from a parent's unrealistic expectations regarding a youngster's abilities in academic, social, or emotional functioning. For example, emphasis may be placed on a separation-anxious youngster's chronological age (e.g., "You're 15 years old—you *should* be able to stay home alone") rather than his or her coping abilities. If such out-of-sync expectations are negatively affecting treatment outcome, consider administering our Parental Expectancies Scale (PES; Eisen et al., 2004; see Appendix I). Sample items include "I expect my child to receive better grades than he/she currently does" and "I expect my child to increase the quality and/or quantity of his/her friendships." The PES will help you determine the extent to which cognitive and educational interventions for parents are needed.

Finally, if significant parental psychopathology (e.g., depression, anxiety, marital conflict) is evident, caregivers may need to seek treatment for their own issues as a first step (see Chapters 3 and 6).

CONSIDERING PHARMACOTHERAPY

Using pharmacotherapy with children and adolescents continues to be a controversial issue. Although advances have emerged in the treatment of childhood anxiety disorders, uncertainties remain regarding medication efficacy, safety, toxicity, and the adequacies of clinical services (Walkup, Labellarte, & Ginsburg, 2002).

Pharmacotherapy is rarely utilized for youngsters with separation anxiety. Medications may be needed, however, for comorbid problems such as chronic school refusal behavior, depression, and OCD. In the next section, we discuss the pharmacotherapy of separation anxiety and related problems. We focus on controlled clinical trials with tricyclic antidepressants (TCAs), selective serotonin reuptake inhibitors (SSRIs), and benzodiazepines (BZDs).

Tricyclic Antidepressants

A limited number of controlled studies has examined the treatment of separation anxiety with tricyclic antidepressants (TCAs) (Bernstein, Borchardt, et al., 2000; Bernstein, Garfinkel, & Borchardt, 1990; Bernstein, Hektner, Borchardt, & McMillan, 2001; Gittelman-Klein & Klein, 1980; Klein, Koplewicz, & Kanner, 1992). Overall, data suggest equivocal therapeutic effects for imipramine (IMI [Tofranil]).

In the first double-blind placebo-controlled trial with youngsters (ages 6–14 years) exhibiting school refusal behavior (93% experienced separation anxiety), Gittelman-Klein and Klein (1980) found evidence supporting the therapeutic efficacy of IMI. For example, child, parent, and clinician ratings demonstrated improvements regarding somatic complaints, fearfulness, and separation anxiety (100% for IMI vs. 21% for placebo). In addition, 81% of youngsters treated with IMI returned to school, compared to 47% of the youngsters on placebo.

The promise of antidepressant treatment has not been realized in other investigations. For example, in a carefully defined sample of youngsters meeting diagnostic criteria for SAD, Klein and colleagues (1992) found that IMI showed no significant superiority compared to placebo, based on child, parent, teacher, and clinical ratings.

Most recently, the combination of IMI and cognitive-behavioral therapy in a sample of adolescents with school refusal behavior, anxiety, and/or depression was investigated (Bernstein, Borchardt, et al., 2000). The results demonstrated that 54% and 17% returned to school for the IMI and placebo groups, respectively. However, 64% of the participants still met criteria for an anxiety disorder at 1-year follow-up (Bernstein et al., 2001). The data suggest an important role for cognitive-behavioral therapy in the treatment of school refusal behavior.

Overall, the therapeutic efficacy of TCAs for separation anxiety and related problems is mixed. In addition, potentially serious side effects, including cardiovascular (e.g., tachycardia), anticholinergic (e.g., dizziness), and central nervous system (e.g., seizures) symptoms, have been well documented (Ambrosini, Bianchi, Rabinovich, & Elia, 1993; Simeon & Wiggins, 1995). As a result, there has been movement toward the use of SSRIs for childhood anxiety disorders due to greater efficacy and safety (e.g., Walkup et al., 2002).

Selective Serotonin Reuptake Inhibitors

In an early double-blind study of youngsters ages 9–14 years with school refusal behavior (87% had separation anxiety), Berney and colleagues (1981) found that the TCA clomipramine (which is a serotonin reuptake inhibitor) was not superior to a placebo.

Greater promise has been realized for selective serotonin reuptake inhibitors (SSRIs). For example, Birmaher and colleagues (1994) demonstrated the efficacy of fluoxetine (Prozac) for children and adolescents (ages 9–18 years) with generalized anxiety, social phobia (SOP), or SAD. Participants were treated openly with fluoxetine for up to 10 months. Eighty-one percent of the participants showed moderate-to-marked improvement, with minimal side effects, on clinician, parent, and child ratings of anxiety.

Further support for the efficacy of fluoxetine was demonstrated in a controlled study of 74 children and adolescents with GAD, SAD, or SOP. Following the 12-week trial, 61% (drug) and 35% (placebo) were considered much improved based on clinician ratings. Side effects were mild and transient and included stomachaches and headaches (Birmaher et al., 2003).

Fluvoxamine (Luvox) is also gaining support as an effective agent in the treatment of anxious youth. Following an 8-week controlled trial of 128 children and adolescents (with SAD, SOP, or GAD), 76% (drug) and 29% (placebo) were considered improved on clinician ratings. The medication was well tolerated in both groups. For example, only 8% (drug) and 2% (placebo) of the participants had to discontinue treatment due to side effects or lack of therapeutic efficacy (Research Units of Psychopharmacology; RUPP, 2001).

Benzodiazepines

Because of their anxiolytic properties, benzodiazepines are sometimes considered in the treatment of anxious youth. However, potentially serious side effects, including addiction, disinhibition, and agitation, have limited their use (Velosa & Riddle, 2000). Of the small number of studies conducted, no demonstrated efficacy has been established for alprazolam (Xanax) in the treatment of school refusal behavior (Bernstein et al., 1990) and generalized anxiety (Simeon et al., 1992), or clonazepam (Klonopin) for SAD (Graae, Milner, Rizzotto, & Klein, 1994).

The nonbenzodiazepine anxiolytic buspirone (BuSpar) has shown promise in the treatment of anxious youth and has less potential for dependence and abuse (Simeon & Wiggins, 1995). However, data demonstrating its therapeutic efficacy are limited to open, uncontrolled trials (e.g., Simeon et al., 1994).

Summary of Pharmacological Studies

Overall, the pharmacotherapy of separation anxiety is extremely limited. Most studies are hampered by methodological constraints, including small sample sizes, diagnostic heterogeneity, and an absence of placebo controls. Given the lack of established guidelines regarding drug treatment for anxiety disorders and data demonstrating long-term safety and efficacy, there has been movement toward an evidenced-based medicine model (Sackett, Richardson, Rosenberg, & Haynes, 2000). Multisite combined treatment efforts (i.e., drug and cognitive-behavioral therapy) are currently underway for a range of internalizing and externalizing disorders (see March, 2002), to set the stage for prescribing specific treatment interventions (i.e., drug, cognitive-behavioral therapy, drug plus cognitive-behavioral therapy), based on a youngster's individual characteristics. Until this model is realized, cognitive-behavioral therapy should be utilized as a first course of action when treating youngsters with separation anxiety and related problems. When anxiety symptoms remain severe and chronic and drug treatment is recommended, SSRIs appear to be the drug class of choice (Pine, 2002).

TERMINATION ISSUES

Once treatment goals have been reached, our next objective is to address termination issues. Important areas to cover may include:

- Reviewing progress in the context of treatment outcome expectancies
- Addressing mixed emotions regarding termination
- Identifying posttreatment goals

In each of the cases described in this volume, youngsters made appropriate and expected progress, and families were generally satisfied with treatment outcomes. It's important to remember, however, that some family members may remain disenchanted regarding a youngster's degree of progress. If a family concludes therapy feeling dissatisfied with the program, maintenance and generalization of treatment gains may suffer. For this reason, we emphasize to parents that skill building takes time to learn, and that some youngsters may simply require more time than others to master the skills. Thus, future improvement is likely with continued practice (Eisen & Kearney, 1995).

In addition to addressing treatment outcome expectancies, separation-anxious youth and their parents may experience a range of emotions during the process of termination. For example, children with intense attachments are more likely to experience fear and sadness as the termination process emerges. In some cases, a child may view you as part of his or her family and have difficulty understanding why continued visits will soon cease. This reaction is especially likely for youngsters who have abandonment issues. Under such circumstances, consider gradually tapering off the sessions (i.e., every other week, once a month) until the youngster becomes accustomed to meeting with you on a periodic basis. At that point, termination can be framed as a *break* from treatment and left open for the possibility of future sessions, as needed.

Older children and adolescents are more likely to experience either eagerness or ambivalence regarding termination. Eagerness may stem from a youngster's view that he or she was coerced into participating in your program. Now that treatment has *finally* concluded, his or her efforts are no longer required. As you can imagine, Natalie was dismayed about having to continue with the program over the summer.

Ambivalence regarding termination is frequently characteristic of adolescents who have behaviorally inhibited temperaments. This response is not surprising, given that ambivalence has been expressed throughout the treatment process. Although the youngster understands the rationale for conducting exposures, he or she still exerts passive resistance. This response was certainly evident in Felicia. Upon termination, Felicia expressed relief that exposures would be less regular. However, she remained uncertain as to whether she was fully prepared to cope on her own (i.e., at sleepaway camp).

Similarly, parents of separation-anxious youth may also experience a gamut of emotions during the termination process. Most typically, however, are relief that the hard work is over and/or apprehension that future treatment sessions may be needed. Providing reassurances regarding posttreatment planning and relapse prevention (to be discussed) can easily allay these insecurities.

Transfer of Control

During treatment, you have taught the child and/or the parent coping skills, provided structure, and helped set and enforce limits during exposure-based homework assignments. As a result, family members may give you undue credit for promoting positive treatment outcomes. At termination, however, be sure to make it clear that your role was that of a facilitator. After all, the efforts of the youngster and parent(s) during treatment were responsible for therapeutic progress. Express confidence in the family's greater abilities to address events associated with separation-anxious responses. Because of those abilities, your guidance is no longer as necessary. Hence, you are "transferring control" to the family so that they can be held responsible for a youngster's continued progress (Silverman & Kurtines, 1996b).

Create the expectation that with regular practice of prescriptive coping skills, continued progress is inevitable. This sustained practice can be accomplished by encouraging youngsters to challenge themselves with posttreatment goals. For example, although Brian was sleeping through the night, he still needed his "blankie." Naturally the idea was not to *discard* the "blankie" he'd had from birth (no matter how shredded), but to minimize his perception that it was needed to help him cope. We suggested that he find a special place for its storage, at least initially, in plain view (e.g., shelf, closet with door open). Then it could be placed out of sight to further enhance his perception of control.

Similarly, Michael was also sleeping through the night toward the end of the treatment program. However, he was still allowed to make one emergency call to his mother from his walkie-talkie. We encouraged him to gradually give up his emergency call, followed by ultimately relinquishing his walkie-talkie. As you can imagine, his mother was not to keen with this suggestion due to his probable resistance. We explained that continued challenges on Michael's part would minimize the likelihood of slips. She didn't even want to think about that possibility. Nevertheless, relapse prevention is an important part of the therapeutic process.

RELAPSE PREVENTION

The process of behavior change is three-pronged:

- Making a commitment to change
- Working through resistance
- Maintaining treatment goals

The first goal is no easy task. Many families *think about* helping their youngsters to change. Far fewer, however, actually have the courage to make the commitment that is necessary to implement lasting change. This ambivalence is often expressed during the initial phone screen or parent consultation.

As you know, the second goal can be quite a challenge as well. However, the families that readily make the commitment up-front are the most likely to follow through in the end. Of course, the road may be bumpy at times, which is why we have armed you with an arsenal of strategies with which to help families realize their goals.

Comparatively, *maintaining* treatment goals should be the most straightforward part of the therapeutic process. This is true for some families. For others, however, the tendency to slip back into previous patterns (without your guidance) or to overreact to setbacks warrants a plan for relapse prevention. In the next section, we discuss expectation of slips, preparing for them, and recovering from them.

Slip Expectation

Once transfer of control has occurred, the process of relapse prevention begins with helping children and their families *expect* and *accept* the possibility of slips. We refer to slips as isolated incidents of backsliding (Marlatt, 1985). Most separation-anxious youngsters will continue to experience some residual anxiety. A family's reaction to a slip, however, is of crucial importance. Catastrophic reactions (e.g., "We'll have to start all over") may lead to relapse or a full-blown return of previous separation-anxious symptoms. To preclude this outcome, be sure to explain the following points to children and their families (Kendall, 1990):

- Everyone slips.
- Slips are part of the learning process.
- Slips are due to relaxed efforts (i.e., lack of practicing prescriptive coping skills).
- Continued practice minimizes the frequency and intensity of slips.

Slip Preparation

The next step of relapse prevention is to help prepare youngsters and their parents for specific "slip scenarios." For example, given Montana's reflux condition, it would not be surprising for her to vomit during the follow-up period, especially if she were stressed. As a first step, we encouraged Mrs. W. to attempt to manage Montana's slips on her own. Specific treatment strategies were discussed as well as a need for phone consultations. At the same time, however, a booster session (to be discussed) was scheduled in 1 month's time. Finally, we discussed the possibility that Montana could attend sessions at a later time if other problems emerged in the future.

For older children and adolescents, imaginal exposures regarding expected slips can be useful. Given that sleepaway camp was 3 months away, we had Felicia (1) imagine, in vivid detail, worst-case scenarios involving social, eating, and interoceptive (e.g., hyperventilation) situations; (2) rate her anxiety on a 0–10 scale; and (3) indicate when the exposure became overwhelming. As her anxiety peaked (6 or more), we encouraged her to practice prescriptive coping skills. Once she habituated to her anxiety (rating of 3 or less), we moved to the next item. When Felicia expressed relative confidence that she could handle the camp experience, we set up a booster session 2 weeks prior to the beginning of camp to review skills and develop an action plan to ensure success.

At the end of the summer, Felicia and her parents were pleased to report that her camp experience was overwhelmingly positive. Six months later, however, a disgruntled Felicia returned for an unplanned follow-up visit. She had recently experienced her first limited-symptom *uncued* panic attack. As a result, she was losing her awareness of all of her accomplishments: "Why does this keep happening to me? I'll never be normal." It was the perfect time to review her slip-recovery exercises.

Slip Recovery

To minimize the frequency and intensity of slips and a family's premature return for continued treatment, consider using any of the following strategies:

- Compile a scrapbook of successful coping reminders (photographs, DD entries, contingency contracts; Kearney & Albano, 2000).
- Film a videotaped infomercial of the youngster as expert explaining how he or she coped with separation anxiety (Kendall et al., 1992).
- Film a videotaped therapy session in which you review prescriptive coping skills, transfer control, and discuss posttreatment goals.
- Record an audiocassette of a therapy session.
- Prepare child and parent slipping handouts that describe a healthy view of slips, how to practice prescriptive coping skills, and how to conduct specific exposures (Eisen & Kearney, 1995).

To minimize the frequency and intensity of slips, encourage children and their families to review these materials periodically and during any anticipated stressors.

Regarding Felicia, we spent a session reviewing slip recovery exercises as well as discussing her remarkable posttreatment progress. We reframed her limited-symptom panic attack as a function of her relaxed coping efforts during the follow-up period. In fact, this was her only episode of anxiety in the last 9 months. To monitor her progress, we scheduled booster sessions at 3- and 6-month intervals.

Booster Sessions

As the treatment program concludes, we always leave the door open for planned or spontaneous (as needed) booster sessions. Remember, our goal is to help *manage* rather than cure a youngster's separation anxiety and related problems (Kendall, 2000). Be sure to explain that returning for periodic visits is expected and *not* a sign of weakness or failure. In fact, failure to return for booster sessions may leave some youngsters feeling ashamed that they let everyone down.

Follow-up periods are regularly scheduled at 1-, 3-, and 6-month intervals and typically involve some form of treatment (e.g., Eisen & Kearney, 1995), such as:

- Praising families continued efforts and accomplishments.
- Reframing slips and reviewing relapse prevention exercises.
- Reviewing prescriptive coping skills.
- Coordinating additional exposure-based homework assignments.
- Planning for anticipated transitions or stressors.

If spontaneous slips occur prior to scheduled booster sessions, consider telephone consultations and office visits, as needed.

Following her second planned booster session, Felicia did not demonstrate any further panic symptoms. Her previous treatment (and maintenance efforts) may have averted the development of uncued panic attacks.

The Nature of Relapse

In general, full-blown relapses rarely occur in anxious youth following successful cognitive-behavioral treatment (Kendall, Safford, Flannery-Schroeder, & Webb, 2004). More specifically, SAD has an extremely high rate of recovery. For example, in one study, 96% of the treated children and adolescents no longer met diagnostic criteria during the follow-up period (Last, Perrin, Hersen, & Kazdin, 1996). Prognosis is poor, however, for youngsters who remain untreated (e.g., Dadds et al., 1999).

Slips are common and may occur as the result of anticipated transitions (e.g., beginning of school year), unexpected stressors (e.g., family illness) or relaxed coping efforts during the follow-up period. In our experience, the majority of youngsters will negotiate separation anxiety, but may retain features of comorbid disorders, especially those of generalized anxiety. For example, in one study symptoms of generalized anxiety were still present in almost half the sample of anxious youth during a 2.5-year follow-up interval (Cohen et al., 1993). In a later study, youngsters with GAD at intake were most likely to develop new emotional disorders (e.g., panic, major depression) during a 9-year follow-up interval (Pine, Cohen, Gurley, Brook, & Ma, 1998). Longer and more routine follow-up intervals may be needed when comorbid symptoms of generalized anxiety are chronic or severe.

SUMMARY

Separation anxiety disorder is the most common anxiety disorder experienced by children and adolescents. Given the diagnostic limitations of DSM-IV and the frequent comorbidity of SAD, we presented an alternative approach to assessing and treating separation-anxious youth that is both dimensional (FBA, FAb, FPI, and WCE) and prescriptive (i.e., matches specific client characteristics with most compatible treatments). Cognitive-behavioral therapy has proven to be remarkably effective in the treatment of anxious youth, in general, and those with separation anxiety, in particular. The merits of pharmacotherapy, however, remain uncertain and appear more appropriate for challenging comorbid disorders. Finally, the relationship between separation anxiety and panic remains unclear. It is our hope that an emphasis on separation-anxiety symptom dimensions will help unravel the pathways to panic and facilitate preventive efforts in separation-anxious youth.

ASSESSMENT INSTRUMENTS

SEPARATION ANXIETY ASSESSMENT SCALE—
CHILD AND ADOLESCENT VERSION

Name: _____ Age: _____ Date: _____

Directions: Read each question below carefully and decide if it is *never, sometimes, most of the time,* or *all the time* true for you. Then for each question, put an *X* on the line in front of the word that seems to describe you best. There are no right or wrong answers. Remember, choose the word that seems to describe how you usually feel.

How often . . .

1. do you need your mom or dad to stay with you in your bedroom to help you go to sleep at night? __Never __Sometimes __Most of the time __All the time

2. do you visit the nurse or a special teacher at school because you feel sick? __Never __Sometimes __Most of the time __All the time

3. do you worry about getting picked up late from school, a party, or another activity? __Never __Sometimes __Most of the time __All the time

4. are you afraid to be left at home with a babysitter? __Never __Sometimes __Most of the time __All the time

5. has a parent, family member, friend, or relative been in a serious accident? __Never __Sometimes (once) __Most of the time (twice) __All the time (three or more)

(continued)

Developed by Andrew R. Eisen, PhD, Lisa Hahn, Jennifer Hajinlian, Breanna Winder, and Donna B. Pincus, PhD, of the Child Anxiety Disorders Clinic, Fairleigh Dickinson University, and Boston University Center for Anxiety and Related Disorders.
    Investigators interested in using this scale should contact Andrew R. Eisen, PhD, at FDU Child Anxiety Disorders Clinic, 131 Temple Avenue, Hackensack, NJ 07601.

6. do you need your mom or dad to promise to pick you up on time, so that you can go to a play date, birthday party, or after-school activity?   __Never __Sometimes __Most of the time __All the time

7. are you afraid to be alone in your living/family room?   __Never __Sometimes __Most of the time __All the time

8. are you afraid to go to school if you feel sick?   __Never __Sometimes __Most of the time __All the time

9. do you worry about bombings happening in the United States?   __Never __Sometimes __Most of the time __All the time

10. do you need your mom or dad to promise to stay at home so that you can go to a play date, birthday party, or after-school activity?   __Never __Sometimes __Most of the time __All the time

11. has a parent, family member, friend, or relative had a serious illness or died?   __Never __Sometimes (once) __Most of the time (twice) __All the time (three or more)

12. are you afraid to go on a play date at a new friend's house?   __Never __Sometimes __Most of the time __All the time

13. are you afraid to sleep alone at night?   __Never __Sometimes __Most of the time __All the time

14. do you worry about natural disasters such as earthquakes, hurricanes, or floods?   __Never __Sometimes __Most of the time __All the time

15. do you need your mom or dad to stay with you so that you can go on a play date, birthday party, or after-school activity?   __Never __Sometimes __Most of the time __All the time

16. have there been burglaries in your neighborhood?   __Never __Sometimes (once) __Most of the time (twice) __All the time (three or more)

(continued)

17. are you afraid to go on   __Never __Sometimes __Most of the time __All the time
a play date because
you may feel sick?

18. do you need to call   __Never __Sometimes __Most of the time __All the time
your mom or dad so
that you can stay home
with a babysitter?

19. do you follow your mom   __Never __Sometimes __Most of the time __All the time
or dad around the
house?

20. are you afraid to take   __Never __Sometimes __Most of the time __All the time
the bus to school or
camp?

21. do you worry that bad   __Never __Sometimes __Most of the time __All the time
things will happen to
you?

22. do you need to call   __Never __Sometimes __Most of the time __All the time
your mom or dad to
help you stay all night
at a sleep-over?

23. have you heard about   __Never __Sometimes __Most of the time __All the time
or seen bad things   (once)   (twice)   (three or
happening to other   more)
people?

24. are you afraid to be left   __Never __Sometimes __Most of the time __All the time
alone in the bathroom
to brush your teeth or
take a bath/shower?

25. are you afraid to stay at   __Never __Sometimes __Most of the time __All the time
home with a babysitter
while your mom or dad
leaves the house to run
an errand?

26. do you worry that bad   __Never __Sometimes __Most of the time __All the time
things will happen to
your parents?

27. are you afraid to eat   __Never __Sometimes __Most of the time __All the time
lunch at school
because you may throw
up or choke?

28. do you need a   __Never __Sometimes __Most of the time __All the time
nightlight, radio, or
television to help you
go to sleep at night?

(continued)

237

29. has a parent, family member, friend, or teacher been hurt in a natural disaster such as a flood or hurricane? __Never __Sometimes (once) __Most of the time (twice) __All the time (three or more)

30. are you afraid to be alone in your bedroom during the day? __Never __Sometimes __Most of the time __All the time

31. are you afraid to eat breakfast at home because you may throw up or choke? __Never __Sometimes __Most of the time __All the time

32. do you need help from a nurse or special teacher to go to or stay at school? __Never __Sometimes __Most of the time __All the time

33. are you afraid to be dropped off at a best friend's house for a play date? __Never __Sometimes __Most of the time __All the time

34. do you need a special blanket or toy to help you feel safe when leaving your house? __Never __Sometimes __Most of the time __All the time

(continued)

SAAS-C SCORING SHEET

To score the SAAS-C, record the numerical response to each question for the subtypes below. A response of *never* = 1, *sometimes* = 2, *most of the time* = 3, and *all the time* = 4. Total each subtype column and compute the average for each subtype. Rank order the subtypes at the bottom of the sheet. SSI = safety signals index.

FBA		FCE	
7.	_____	5.	_____
13.	_____	11.	_____
19.	_____	16.	_____
24.	_____	23.	_____
30.	_____	29.	_____
Total:	_____	Total:	_____
Avg.:	_____	Avg.:	_____

FAb		WCE	
4.	_____	3.	_____
12.	_____	9.	_____
20.	_____	14.	_____
25.	_____	21.	_____
33.	_____	26.	_____
Total:	_____	Total:	_____
Avg.:	_____	Avg.:	_____

FPI		SSI	
2.	_____	1.	_____
8.	_____	6.	_____
17.	_____	10.	_____
27.	_____	15.	_____
31.	_____	18.	_____
		22.	_____
Total:	_____	28.	_____
Avg.:	_____	32.	_____
		34.	_____
		Total:	_____
		Avg.:	_____

RANK: 1._____ 2._____ 3._____ 4._____ 5._____

SSI Total Score: _____

239

SEPARATION ANXIETY ASSESSMENT SCALE— PARENT VERSION

Name: _____ Age: _____ Date: _____

Directions: Read each question below carefully and decide if it is *never*, *sometimes*, *most of the time*, or *all the time* true for your child. Then for each question, put an *X* on the line in front of the word that seems to describe him or her best. There are no right or wrong answers. Remember, choose the word that seems to describe how your child usually feels.

How often . . .

1. do you need to stay in your child's bedroom to help him or her go to sleep at night? __Never __Sometimes __Most of the time __All the time

2. does your child visit the nurse or a special teacher at school because he or she feels sick? __Never __Sometimes __Most of the time __All the time

3. does your child verbalize worries about getting picked up late from school, a party, or another activity? __Never __Sometimes __Most of the time __All the time

4. is your child afraid to be left at home with a babysitter? __Never __Sometimes __Most of the time __All the time

5. have you, a family member, friend, or relative been in a serious accident? __Never __Sometimes (once) __Most of the time (twice) __All the time (three or more)

(continued)

Developed by Andrew R. Eisen, PhD, Lisa Hahn, Jennifer Hajinlian, Breanna Winder, and Donna B. Pincus, PhD, of the Child Anxiety Disorders Clinic, Fairleigh Dickinson University, and Boston University Center for Anxiety and Related Disorders.
Investigators using this scale should contact: Andrew R. Eisen, PhD, at FDU Child Anxiety Disorders Clinic, 131 Temple Avenue, Hackensack, NJ 07601.

6. do you need to promise to pick up your child on time, so he or she can go to a play date, birthday party, or after-school activity? __Never __Sometimes __Most of the time __All the time

7. is your child afraid to be alone in your living/family room? __Never __Sometimes __Most of the time __All the time

8. is your child afraid to go to school if he or she feels sick? __Never __Sometimes __Most of the time __All the time

9. does your child verbalize worries about bombings happening in the United States? __Never __Sometimes __Most of the time __All the time

10. do you need to promise to stay at home so your child can go to a play date, birthday party, or after-school activity? __Never __Sometimes __Most of the time __All the time

11. have you, a family member, friend, or relative had a serious illness? __Never __Sometimes (once) __Most of the time (twice) __All the time (three or more)

12. is your child afraid to go on a play date at a new friend's house? __Never __Sometimes __Most of the time __All the time

13. is your child afraid to sleep alone at night? __Never __Sometimes __Most of the time __All the time

14. does your child verbalize worries about natural disasters such as hurricanes or floods? __Never __Sometimes __Most of the time __All the time

15. do you need to stay with your child so he or she can go on a play date, birthday party, or after-school activity? __Never __Sometimes __Most of the time __All the time

16. have there been burglaries in your neighborhood? __Never __Sometimes (once) __Most of the time (twice) __All the time (three or more)

(continued)

17. is your child afraid to go on a play date because he or she may feel sick?   __Never __Sometimes __Most of the time __All the time

18. does your child need to call you so that he or she can stay with a babysitter?   __Never __Sometimes __Most of the time __All the time

19. does your child follow you around the house?   __Never __Sometimes __Most of the time __All the time

20. is your child afraid to take the bus to school or camp?   __Never __Sometimes __Most of the time __All the time

21. does your child verbalize worries that bad things will happen to him or her?   __Never __Sometimes __Most of the time __All the time

22. does your child need to call you so that he or she can stay all night at a sleep-over?   __Never __Sometimes __Most of the time __All the time

23. has your child heard about or seen bad things happening to other people?   __Never __Sometimes (once) __Most of the time (twice) __All the time (three or more)

24. is your child afraid to be left alone in the bathroom to brush his or her teeth or take a bath/shower?   __Never __Sometimes __Most of the time __All the time

25. is your child afraid to stay home with a babysitter while you leave the house to run an errand?   __Never __Sometimes __Most of the time __All the time

26. does your child verbalize worries that bad things will happen to you?   __Never __Sometimes __Most of the time __All the time

27. is your child afraid to eat lunch at school because he or she may throw up or choke?   __Never __Sometimes __Most of the time __All the time

(continued)

242

28. does your child need a nightlight, radio, or television to help him or her go to sleep at night? __Never __Sometimes __Most of the time __All the time

29. have you, a family member, friend, or teacher been hurt in a natural disaster such as a flood or hurricane? __Never __Sometimes (once) __Most of the time (twice) __All the time (three or more)

30. is your child afraid to be alone in his or her bedroom during the day? __Never __Sometimes __Most of the time __All the time

31. is your child afraid to eat breakfast at home because he or she may throw up or choke? __Never __Sometimes __Most of the time __All the time

32. does your child need help from a nurse or special teacher to go to or stay at school? __Never __Sometimes __Most of the time __All the time

33. is your child afraid to be dropped off at a best friend's house for a play date? __Never __Sometimes __Most of the time __All the time

34. does your child need a special blanket/toy to help him or her feel safe when leaving the house? __Never __Sometimes __Most of the time __All the time

(continued)

SAAS-P SCORING SHEET

To score the SAAS-P, record the numerical response to each question for the subtypes below. A response of *never* = 1, *sometimes* = 2, *most of the time* = 3, and *all the time* = 4. Total each subtype column and compute the average for each subtype. Rank order the subtypes at the bottom of the sheet. SSI = safety signals index.

FBA		FCE	
7.	_____	5.	_____
13.	_____	11.	_____
19.	_____	16.	_____
24.	_____	23.	_____
30.	_____	29.	_____
Total:	_____	Total:	_____
Avg.:	_____	Avg.:	_____

FAb		WCE	
4.	_____	3.	_____
12.	_____	9.	_____
20.	_____	14.	_____
25.	_____	21.	_____
33.	_____	26.	_____
Total:	_____	Total:	_____
Avg.:	_____	Avg.:	_____

FPI		SSI	
2.	_____	1.	_____
8.	_____	6.	_____
17.	_____	10.	_____
27.	_____	15.	_____
31.	_____	18.	_____
		22.	_____
Total:	_____	28.	_____
Avg.:	_____	32.	_____
		34.	_____
		Total:	_____
		Avg.:	_____

RANK: 1. _____   2. _____   3. _____   4. _____   5. _____

SSI Total Score: _____

In the following tables, we present some preliminary norms for SAAS-C and SAAS-P dimensions. We compare separation anxiety disorder (SAD) to other anxiety disorders (e.g., GAD, social and specific phobias) and externalizing disorders (e.g., ADHD, ODD).

SAAS-C Norms across DSM-IV Diagnostic Categories

SAAS-C (mean)	Diagnosis		
	SAD	Other anxiety	Externalizing
FBA	11.0	6.9	10.5
FAb	12.0	6.3	7.0
FPI	9.5	7.9	9.5
WCE	13.5	8.8	10.5
FCE	8.0	7.4	7.0
SSI	22.0	12.2	16.5
Total	75.0	49.5	60.0

SAAS-P Norms Across DSM-IV Diagnostic Categories

SAAS-C (mean)	Diagnosis		
	SAD	Other anxiety	Externalizing
FBA	11.0	7.6	8.0
FAb	10.0	7.8	6.0
FPI	8.5	8.3	5.8
WCE	11.0	9.8	6.7
FCE	6.5	6.7	5.2
SSI	16.0	11.9	11.5
Total	64.0	52.1	43.4

PARENTAL EXPECTANCIES SCALE

Parent Name: _____

Child's Name: _____

Child's Age: _____ Date: _____

The following are statements that could be made by any parent. With respect to your child, please indicate to what extent these statements reflect your concerns, perceptions, and expectations as a parent. Please circle the number representing the level to which each statement is "true for you." Please do not leave any statement unanswered.

0	1	2	3	4	5
Never or almost never true	Seldom true	Sometimes true	True more often than not	Usually true	Almost always or always true

1. I expect academic success will be an important goal for my child.

   0   1   2   3   4   5

2. Concerning extracurricular activities such as athletics, dance, music instruction, or other organized hobbies, I expect my child to always do his or her best.

   0   1   2   3   4   5

3. I expect my child to pursue only those activities at which he or she can excel.

   0   1   2   3   4   5

4. I expect that popularity and an active social life will be important goals for my child.

   0   1   2   3   4   5

5. I expect my child to receive better grades than he or she currently does.

   0   1   2   3   4   5

6. I expect my child to become more responsible and self-sufficient in home-related activities.

   0   1   2   3   4   5

(continued)

Developed by Andrew R. Eisen, PhD, Sheila A. Spasaro, PhD, and Lisa K. Brien, PhD, Christopher A. Kearney, PhD, and Anne Marie Albano, PhD, of the Child Anxiety Disorders Clinic, Fairleigh Dickinson University; University of Nevada Las Vegas; and NYU Child Study Center.

Investigators interested in using this assessment instrument should contact Andrew R. Eisen, PhD, at FDU Child Anxiety Disorders Clinic, 131 Temple Avenue, Hackensack, NJ 07601.

7. I expect to play an important role in helping my child to socialize, establish new friendships, and maintain current friendships.

    0   1   2   3   4   5

8. I expect my child to perform better in his or her extracurricular activities, such as athletics, dance, music instruction, art instruction, or other organized hobbies.

    0   1   2   3   4   5

9. I expect that experiences of success will be the best reinforcers for my child's self-confidence.

    0   1   2   3   4   5

10. I expect my child to increase the quality and/or quantity of his or her friendships.

    0   1   2   3   4   5

11. I expect my child to participate in many extracurricular activities, such as athletics, dance, music instruction, or other organized hobbies.

    0   1   2   3   4   5

12. My expectations for my child's peer relations differ from his or her own.

    0   1   2   3   4   5

13. I expect my child to do chores in the home on a regular basis.

    0   1   2   3   4   5

14. I expect my child will achieve his or her full potential in life.

    0   1   2   3   4   5

15. My academic expectations for my child differ from his or her own.

    0   1   2   3   4   5

16. I expect my child will distinguish him- or herself with top performances in his or her extracurricular activities.

    0   1   2   3   4   5

17. Whether a child becomes a successful adult greatly depends upon the guidance and encouragement provided by his or her parents.

    0   1   2   3   4   5

18. I expect my child to take initiative in helping out in the home.

    0   1   2   3   4   5

19. If my child has not received a good grade in school, I always expect him or her to try harder.

    0   1   2   3   4   5

20. I expect my child to exhibit exemplary behavior and be very well-mannered when we have guests in our home.

    0   1   2   3   4   5

(continued)

PES SCORING SHEET

To score the PES, record the numerical response to each question for the subscales below. Total each subscale column and compute the average for each subscale. Rank order the subscales at the bottom of the sheet.

School	Extracurricular	Social	Home	General Success
1 _____	2 _____	4 _____	6 _____	3 _____
5 _____	8 _____	7 _____	13 _____	9 _____
15 _____	11 _____	10 _____	18 _____	14 _____
19 _____	16 _____	12 _____	20 _____	17 _____

Each Column
Total Score

_____   _____   _____   _____   _____

All Columns
Total Score

_____

Mean Score

_____   _____   _____   _____   _____

Relative Ranking

_____   _____   _____   _____   _____

Norms Based on Total PES Scores (range = 0–100)
70–82: High expectations (unrealistic)
58–69: Realistic expectations (normative)
45–57: Low expectations (parents of anxious youth)

PLAYFULNESS SCALE FOR ADULTS

Instructions: Please respond to the following statements using a 7-point scale to indicate how much you agree with each statement. Indicate **1** for "strongly disagree," **3** for "somewhat disagree," **5** for "somewhat agree," and **7** for "strongly agree."

1. I enjoy acting a bit wild and crazy at times.

Strongly
disagree
1   2   3   4   5   6   Strongly agree 7

2. I consider myself to be a serious, no-nonsense type of a person.

Strongly
disagree
1   2   3   4   5   6   Strongly agree 7

3. I find the daily comic strips amusing.

Strongly
disagree
1   2   3   4   5   6   Strongly agree 7

4. I would like a nerf basketball hoop in my bedroom.

Strongly
disagree
1   2   3   4   5   6   Strongly agree 7

5. I like my day to be tightly structured so I'll know exactly where I'll be and what I'll be doing.

Strongly
disagree
1   2   3   4   5   6   Strongly agree 7

6. I get so competitive during card games or sporting events that they become more work than play to me.

Strongly
disagree
1   2   3   4   5   6   Strongly agree 7

(continued)

Developed by Charles E. Schaefer, PhD, and Robin Greenberg, MA, Department of Psychology, Fairleigh Dickinson University.

Investigators interested in using this assessment instrument should contact Charles E. Schaefer, PhD, at Department of Psychology, Fairleigh Dickinson University, 1000 River Road, Teaneck, NJ 07666.

7. I enjoy acting silly or goofy at times.

Strongly
disagree

Strongly
agree

1   2   3   4   5   6   7

8. I would rather go to a museum than an amusement park.

Strongly
disagree

Strongly
agree

1   2   3   4   5   6   7

9. At times I'll sing in the shower or do a little dance at home.

Strongly
disagree

Strongly
agree

1   2   3   4   5   6   7

10. I like to find ways to have fun at work.

Strongly
disagree

Strongly
agree

1   2   3   4   5   6   7

11. I would rather read a book than play a game.

Strongly
disagree

Strongly
agree

1   2   3   4   5   6   7

12. I find it hard to laugh at myself.

Strongly
disagree

Strongly
agree

1   2   3   4   5   6   7

13. I would rather go to Toys R Us than browse at the mall.

Strongly
disagree

Strongly
agree

1   2   3   4   5   6   7

14. I think life is more like a comedy than a tragedy.

Strongly
disagree

Strongly
agree

1   2   3   4   5   6   7

15. If I'm feeling blue, laughing tends to make me feel better.

Strongly
disagree

Strongly
agree

1   2   3   4   5   6   7

16. Winning is everything when playing a game.

Strongly
disagree

Strongly
agree

1   2   3   4   5   6   7

(continued)

17. To me, clowning or playing around is more a waste of time than anything else.

Strongly
disagree

Strongly
agree

1   2   3   4   5   6   7

18. Even the most serious situation is likely to have a funny side to it.

Strongly
disagree

Strongly
agree

1   2   3   4   5   6   7

19. I like to smile and laugh as much as possible during the day.

Strongly
disagree

Strongly
agree

1   2   3   4   5   6   7

20. I usually don't enjoy jokes or playful teasing.

Strongly
disagree

Strongly
agree

1   2   3   4   5   6   7

21. I'm usually one of the first to initiate fun activities when I'm with my friends.

Strongly
disagree

Strongly
agree

1   2   3   4   5   6   7

22. I would much rather accept a job that is personally enjoyable than one with a wonderful salary.

Strongly
disagree

Strongly
agree

1   2   3   4   5   6   7

23. I would never leave work early to do fun activities.

Strongly
disagree

Strongly
agree

1   2   3   4   5   6   7

24. Wearing a mask/costume on Halloween is fun to me.

Strongly
disagree

Strongly
agree

1   2   3   4   5   6   7

25. I still consider it fun to throw snowballs or build sandcastles.

Strongly
disagree

Strongly
agree

1   2   3   4   5   6   7

(continued)

26. I enjoy watching *Star Trek* and other science fiction shows.

Strongly disagree   Strongly agree

1   2   3   4   5   6   7

27. I can't find anything amusing about watching a "Three Stooges" movie.

Strongly disagree   Strongly agree

1   2   3   4   5   6   7

28. At times, I find it fun to play video or computer games.

Strongly disagree   Strongly agree

1   2   3   4   5   6   7

29. I keep a tight rein on my impulses and emotions.

Strongly disagree   Strongly agree

1   2   3   4   5   6   7

30. I like to give and receive cartoon or joke book gifts.

Strongly disagree   Strongly agree

1   2   3   4   5   6   7

31. I'm very comfortable playing with games or toys on the floor with kids.

Strongly disagree   Strongly agree

1   2   3   4   5   6   7

32. My close friends expect lighthearted ribbing from me.

Strongly disagree   Strongly agree

1   2   3   4   5   6   7

33. I never make up silly names for people I care about.

Strongly disagree   Strongly agree

1   2   3   4   5   6   7

34. People consider me a "fun" person.

Strongly disagree   Strongly agree

1   2   3   4   5   6   7

35. I enjoy playing charades.

Strongly disagree   Strongly agree

1   2   3   4   5   6   7

(continued)

PSA SCORING SHEET

To score the PSA, compute a total score by adding each of the numerical items circled. Items 6, 8, 11, 16, 26, 27, and 28 are not included in the total score. Items 2, 5, 6, 8, 11, 12, 16, 17, 20, 23, 27, 29, and 33 are **reverse scored**.

Range is 28–196.

138 (normative)

158 + (high playfulness)

118 and below (low playfulness)

HANDOUTS

Handout I

RELAXATION SCRIPT

1. The Introduction

Okay, [insert child's name], it's time to relax. Close your eyes. Just loosen up all the muscles in your body. Anything that you're thinking about . . . school, family, or friends . . . just push those thoughts away. *This is your time.* Just relax. I want you to listen to the sound of my voice and perform the following exercises. Let's begin . . .

2. Fists

[Insert child's name], this exercise is for your hands and fingers. First, hold your arms out in front of you. Now, make fists with both hands. Squeeze hard. All the tension, all the frustration, all the anxiety—hold it tight in your fists . . . Now relax . . . Open up your hands and let your fingers be loose. Notice the difference, [insert child's name], when your hands are all tight and tense, and when they are nice . . . and loose . . . and relaxed. That's how we want you to feel. Nice . . . and loose . . . and relaxed. Let's try this again . . . First, hold your arms out in front of you. Now, make fists with both hands. Clench your fists hard. Hold them . . . good. Now relax again . . . Just kind of settle down, get comfortable, and relax. You feel good . . . and warm . . . and lazy.

Helpful Things to Say

[Insert child's name], sometimes it's hard to relax. We may be thinking about other things, like school, family, or friends. If you are having trouble relaxing, just do the best you can to push those thoughts away. The more you practice, the easier it will be to relax.

[Insert child's name], sometimes . . . we are afraid to let go. If we let go, we think we might lose control. Actually, if you let go and allow the relaxation to sink in, you will be in *total control* and you will see how wonderful it feels to be relaxed.

(continued)

Progressive relaxation exercises developed by Thomas H. Ollendick, PhD, and Jerome A. Cerny, PhD, of the Department of Psychology, Virginia Polytechnic and State University, and Indiana University.
    Adapted and reprinted from Ollendick and Cerny (1981). Copyright 1981 by Kluwer Academic/ Plenum Publishers.
    Breathing and visualization exercises developed by Andrew R. Eisen, PhD. Copyright 2005 by Andrew R. Eisen.

Reprinted in *Separation Anxiety in Children and Adolescents: An Individualized Approach to Assessment and Treatment* by Andrew R. Eisen and Charles E. Schaefer.

3. Biceps

The next exercise is for your hands and arms. First, hold your arms out to the side. Now, hold your arms up high and show me your muscles. Tense your biceps. Hold them . . . Show me how strong you are . . . much stronger than all the tension and anxiety. Good . . . Now let go and relax . . . Let your arms be loose and feel how nice that is. It feels good to relax . . . Let's try this again. First, hold your arms out to the side. Now, hold your arms up high and show me your muscles. Tense your biceps. Tighter . . . Good . . . Now relax . . . Notice the difference when your arms are all tight and tense, and when they are nice and loose and relaxed. That's how we want your arms to feel. Nice . . . and loose . . . and relaxed. You feel good, and warm, and lazy.

4. Shoulders and Back

The next exercise is for your shoulders. Tense your shoulders. Push them down. Try to touch the ground. Hold in tight . . . Good . . . Now relax . . . Just loosen up your shoulders and bring them back to their natural, comfortable position. That feels so much better. Let's try this again. Tense your shoulders. Push them down. Tighter . . . Great. Now relax . . . *It feels so good to let go.* Notice that when you relax your shoulders, your back relaxes too, and that feels good . . . Just try to relax your whole body. Let yourself get as loose as you can.

Helpful Things to Say

[Insert child's name], you don't have to shoulder the burdens of the world. You just have to do the best that you can. Sometimes we focus too much on our performance. It's easy to feel good about yourself when you are successful, like winning a game or getting a good grade. The hard part is feeling good even when things do not go your way. If you focus on your efforts, you can always feel good, no matter what the outcome. *Take the pressure off.* Just do the best that you can. Remember, [insert child's name], you cannot fail at anything if you keep trying. So focus on your efforts, keep trying, and do your best. This is what I want you to think about when you're tensing your shoulders.

5. Mouth

[Insert child's name], sometimes when we feel tight and tense, we feel it in the mouth, the jaw, or the teeth. If you feel that way, here is an exercise to practice. Press your lips together. Press them hard. Hold them . . . Good. Now relax. *Just let your mouth be loose. It feels so good to let go.* Let's try this again. Press your lips together. Press hard. Hold them . . . Good. Now relax again. *Just let your mouth be loose.* That feels so much better.

6. Forehead

The next exercise is for your forehead. Make wrinkles on your forehead. *Raise your eyebrows.* All the tension, all the frustration, all the anxiety—hold it all in your forehead. Now relax . . . Let your forehead be smooth. Your forehead feels nice and smooth and relaxed. Let's try this again. Make wrinkles on your forehead.

(continued)

Raise your eyebrows. Hold them tight until I count to three. One . . . Two . . . Three . . . Now let it all go. No wrinkles anywhere. Your face feels nice and smooth and relaxed.

7. Mean Face

The next exercise is for your whole face. Scrunch up your face—make wrinkles on your forehead. Raise your eyebrows. Push out your lower jaw. Frown big. *Make a mean face.* Hold it all tight . . . Now relax . . . No more wrinkles. Your face feels nice and smooth and relaxed.

Why did I ask you to make a mean face? Sometimes when we get angry, we say mean things, hurtful things, to the people we care about, like, *I hate you* or *I will never play with you again.* Sometimes we *do* mean things, like pushing people or throwing things when we get upset. [Insert child's name], it would be better to make a *mean face.* No consequences for that. It's a great way of getting rid of your anger.

Let's try it again. *Show me your mean face.* Hold it tight . . . Good. Now relax . . . No wrinkles anywhere. Your face feels nice and smooth and relaxed.

8. Stomach

The next exercise is for your stomach. Tighten up your stomach. Hold it. Don't move . . . Now relax. Just kind of settle down, get comfortable, and relax. Let your stomach come back out where it belongs. That feels so much better. Let's try this again. Tighten up . . . Tighten hard . . . Hold it. Now relax. [Insert child's name], notice the difference between a tight stomach and a relaxed one. That's how we want your stomach to feel. Nice . . . and loose . . . and relaxed. Now you can relax completely.

9. Summary of Exercises

[Insert child's name], let's make sure that all your muscles are nice and loose and relaxed. Your stomach should be resting in its natural, comfortable position. Your whole face is completely smooth. No wrinkles anywhere. No tension in your mouth. No tension in your shoulders. And remember, [insert child's name], you don't have to shoulder the burdens of the world. Just do the best you can. Your hands and arms feel loose and relaxed and your fingers may feel a bit tingly.

10. Breathing Exercises

[Insert child's name], now it's time to practice our breathing exercises. Most people don't know how to breathe to relax. The trick is to first breathe in deeply through your nose. As you breathe in, be sure to fill up your lungs with air and hold that breath until I tell you to breathe out. When I tell you to breathe out, pretend that you are the wind, and blow that tension a mile away. When you breathe in, you breathe in the good energy and when you breathe out, you let go of your fear. Let's practice. Try to stick to my pace.

Let me *see* you breathe in . . . Let me *hear* you breathe out . . . Let me *see* you breathe in . . . Let me *hear* you breathe out. And as you breathe out, pretend that you are the wind, and blow all that tension a mile away [Repeat.]

(continued)

11. Visualization Exercises

[Insert child's name], I want you to keep breathing in through your nose and breathing out through your mouth. At the same time, I want you to pretend that you are stepping aboard a hot-air balloon. As you breathe in and breathe out, you will fill the hot-air balloon, and it will take you wherever you would like to go.

Scene 1

Suddenly, you find yourself high in the sky . . . It's a beautiful spring day . . . The sky is blue . . . You feel the warmth of the sun shining against your forehead . . . A cool breeze blows by [make a gentle swooshing sound] . . . You look down below and see the magnificent forest . . . This is where you go when *you need to relax.*

> Let me *see you* breathe in . . . Let me *hear you* breathe out . . .
> Let me *see you* breathe in . . . Let me *hear you* breathe out . . .
> And as you breathe out, pretend you are the wind and blow the tension a
> mile away.

Scene 2

The hot-air balloon lands on the beach. As you step down, you feel the hot sand against your toes. You see the children swimming in the ocean. The seagulls are flying above you. Just stand there, [insert child's name], and breathe in the ocean air. This is where you go when *you need to relax.*

> Let me *see you* breathe in . . . Let me *hear you* breathe out . . .
> Let me *see you* breathe in . . . Let me *hear you* breathe out . . .
> And as you breathe out, pretend you are the wind and blow the tension a
> mile away.

12. Script Conclusion

Try to stay as relaxed as you can. All your muscles should be nice and loose and relaxed. I want you to listen to this tape every night before you go to bed. You may even fall asleep before the tape is finished. If you listen every night, you will sleep better. You will be calmer. The little things will not bother you as much. But the real trick, [insert child's name], is that I want you to use these exercises in the situations that make you feel scared, like . . . [insert relevant scenarios]. And all you have to do is try your best. And you know what you are going to realize really soon . . . *There is nothing that you cannot do.*

CONTINGENCY CONTRACT

Date: _____

Exposure-based assignment:

_____

_____

_____

Specific conditions:

_____

_____

_____

Relevant details:
(child or adolescent)

DO: (GOAL)

_____

WHAT TO EXPECT (CHILD):

_____

DO: (HOW TO COPE)

_____

Relevant details:
(parent)

DO: (GOAL)

_____

WHAT TO EXPECT (PARENT):

_____

(continued)

DO: (HOW TO HELP CHILD COPE)

_____

_____

REWARD:

Success: _____

_____

Partial success: _____

_____

Relevant signatures:

_____
(Child or Adolescent)

_____
(Parent or Guardian)

_____
(Therapist)

Handout 3

WHAT'S HAPPENING TO ME?

Name: _____   Date: _____

When?	Where?	My Body? (0–10)	My Thoughts? (0–10)	My Feelings? (0–10)

SCALE: (0–1: calm; 2–4: a little uncomfortable; 5–7: uncomfortable; 8–10: very uncomfortable)

COPING WITH MY BODY

Name: _____ Date: _____

When?	Where?	My Body? (0–10)	Relaxation Exercises?	My Body Now? (0–10)	How Did I Cope?	Reward?

SCALE: (0–1: calm; 2–4: a little uncomfortable; 5–7: uncomfortable; 8–10: very uncomfortable)

COPING WITH MY WORRIES

Name: _____   Date: _____

When?	Where?	My Worries? (0–10)	Cognitive Exercises?	My Worries Now? (0–10)	How Did I Cope?	Reward?

SCALE: (0–1: not worried; 2–4: a little worried; 5–7: worried; 8–10: very worried)

WEEKLY RECORD OF ANXIETY AT SEPARATION (WRAS)

The WRAS is a simple and effective way for parents to collect objective data regarding the frequency and intensity of a youngster's separation-anxiety-related behaviors on a daily basis. Cut and paste to provide parents with only the most relevant separation-related situations (e.g., being alone, being abandoned). If situations and/or locations are relevant outside one's home, encourage parent to keep readily available (purse, wallet) to ensure accurate recording. WRAS data will be most helpful when creating exposure hierarchies (see Chapter 8).

Weekly Record of Anxiety at Separation

Please enter the number of times your child engaged in the following behaviors each day in the past week. If your child engaged in the behavior, please rate the amount of distress your child evidenced on a scale from 0 to 8 (0 = no distress, 8 = extremely intense distress).

Separation Anxiety Behaviors	Mon. # Times	Mon. Distress (0–8)	Tues. # Times	Tues. Distress (0–8)	Wed. # Times	Wed. Distress (0–8)	Thurs. # Times	Thurs. Distress (0–8)	Fri. # Times	Fri. Distress (0–8)	Sat. # Times	Sat. Distress (0–8)	Sun. # Times	Sun. Distress (0–8)
Separation Anxiety around School														
Refused to attend school and be away from parent														
Called the parent from school														
Left school early to be with the parent														
Complained of illness to avoid being away from parent														
Separation Anxiety around Bedtime														
Slept in parents' room														
Refused to go to sleep without parent present														
Awakened parents in the night														
Had nightmares involving separation														
Separation Anxiety around Play and Other Activities														
Refused to play without the parent nearby														
Refused to attend or participate in activities (e.g., sports, school outings, games) without the parent nearby														

(continued)

Weekly Record of Anxiety at Separation *(page 2 of 2)*

Separation Anxiety Behaviors	Mon. # Times	Mon. Distress (0–8)	Tues. # Times	Tues. Distress (0–8)	Wed. # Times	Wed. Distress (0–8)	Thurs. # Times	Thurs. Distress (0–8)	Fri. # Times	Fri. Distress (0–8)	Sat. # Times	Sat. Distress (0–8)	Sun. # Times	Sun. Distress (0–8)
Separation Anxiety around Parents' Departure														
Cried/showed distress when anticipating that parent was going to leave														
Complained of illness when anticipating that parent was going to leave														
Cried/showed distress when parents left														
Separation Anxiety around Parents' Location														
Checked on parents' whereabouts during the day/called out to parents, asking where they were														
Followed parents throughout the day														
Avoided being away from parents														
Refused to be alone or without parents														
Separation Anxiety around Parents' Well-Being														
Expressed worry that harm would befall parents														
Expressed worry that something bad might happen to parents														
Separation Anxiety around Child's Well-Being														
Expressed worry that harm would befall child														
Expressed worry that something bad might happen to child														

References

Abidin, R. R. (1995). *Parenting Stress Index (PSI) Manual* (3rd ed.). Odessa, FL: Psychological Assessment Resources.

Achenbach, T. M. (1991a). *Manual for the Child Behavior Checklist/4–18 and 1991 Profile*. Burlington, VT: University of Vermont Department of Psychiatry.

Achenbach, T. M. (1991b). *Manual for the Youth Self-Report and 1991 Profile*. Burlington, VT: University of Vermont Department of Psychiatry.

Ainsworth, M. D. S. (1967). *Infancy in Uganda: Infant care and the growth of love*. Baltimore: Johns Hopkins University Press.

Ainsworth, M. D. S., Blehar, M. C., Waters, E., & Wall, S. (1978). *Patterns of attachment: A psychological study of the strange situation*. Hillsdale, NJ: Erlbaum.

Albano, A. M., & Kendall, P. C. (2002). Cognitive behavioral therapy for children and adolescents with anxiety disorders: Clinical research advances. *International Review of Psychiatry, 14*, 129–134.

Alfven, G. (1993). The covariation of common psychosomatic symptoms among children from socioeconomically differing residential areas: An epidemiological study. *Acta Paediatrica, 82*, 484–487.

Ambrosini, P. J. (2000). Historical development and present status of the Schedule for Affective Disorders and Schizophrenia for School-Age Children (K-SADS). *Journal of the American Academy of Child and Adolescent Psychiatry, 39*, 49–58.

Ambrosini, P. J., Bianchi, M. D., Rabinovich, H., & Elia, J. (1993). Antidepressant treatments in children and adolescents: II. Anxiety, physical and behavioral disorders. *Journal of the American Academy of Child and Adolescent Psychiatry, 32*, 483–493.

American Psychiatric Association. (1994). *Diagnostic and statistical manual of mental disorders* (4th ed.). Washington, DC: Author.

American Psychiatric Association. (2000). *Diagnostic and statistical manual of mental disorders* (4th ed., text rev.). Washington, DC: Author.

Anderson, J. C., Williams, S., McGee, R., & Silva, P. A. (1987). DSM-III disorders in pre-adolescent children: Prevalence in a large sample from the general population. *Archives of General Psychiatry, 44,* 69–76.

Andrews, G. (1995). Comorbidity in neurotic disorders: The similarities are more important than the differences. In R. M. Rapee (Ed.), *Current controversies in the anxiety disorders* (pp. 3–20). New York: Guilford Press.

Angold, A., & Costello, E. J. (2000). The Child and Adolescent Psychiatric Assessment (CAPA). *Journal of the American Academy of Child and Adolescent Psychiatry, 39,* 39–48.

Anthony, J. L., Lonigan, C. J., Hooe, E. S., & Philips, B. M. (2002). An affect-based, hierarchical model of temperament and its relations with internalizing symptomatology. *Journal of Clinical Child and Adolescent Psychology, 31,* 480–490.

Aronen, E. T., & Soininen, M. (2000). Childhood depressive symptoms predict psychiatric problems in young adults. *Canadian Journal of Psychiatry, 45,* 465–470.

Aschenbrand, S. G., Kendall, P. C., Webb, A., Safford, S. M., & Flannery-Schroeder, E. (2003). Is childhood separation anxiety disorder a predictor of adult panic disorder and agoraphobia?: A seven-year longitudinal study. *Journal of the American Academy of Child and Adolescent Psychiatry, 42,* 1478–1485.

Asmundson, G. J., & Stein, M. B. (1994). Triggering the false suffocation alarm in panic disorder patients by using a voluntary breath-holding procedure. *American Journal of Psychiatry, 151,* 264–266.

Ayuso, J., Alfonso, S., & Rivera, A. (1989). Childhood separation anxiety and panic disorder: A comparative study. *Progress in Neuropsychopharmacology and Biological Psychiatry, 13,* 665–671.

Bandura, A. (1988). Self-efficacy conception of anxiety. *Anxiety Research, 1,* 77–98.

Barkley, R. A., Edwards, G. H., & Robin, A. L. (1999). *Defiant teens: A clinician's manual for assessment and family intervention.* New York: Guilford Press.

Barlow, D. H. (1988). *Anxiety and its disorders: The nature and treatment of anxiety and panic.* New York: Guilford Press.

Barlow, D. H. (2002). *Anxiety and its disorders: The nature and treatment of anxiety and panic* (2nd ed.). New York: Guilford Press.

Barrett, P. M., Dadds, M. R., & Rapee, R. M. (1996). Family treatment of childhood anxiety: A controlled trial. *Journal of Consulting and Clinical Psychology, 64*(2), 333–342.

Barrett, P. M., Rapee, R. M., Dadds, M. R., & Ryan, S. M. (1996). Family enhancement of cognitive style in anxious and aggressive children. *Journal of Abnormal Child Psychology, 24,* 187–203.

Barrios, B. A., & Hartmann, D. P. (1997). Fears and anxieties. In E. J. Mash & L. G. Terdal (Eds.), *Assessment of childhood disorders* (3rd ed., pp. 230–237). New York: Guilford Press.

Baumrind, D. (1989). Rearing competent children. In W. Darmon (Ed.), *Child development today and tomorrow* (pp. 349–378). San Francisco, CA: Jossey-Bass.

Beck, A. T. (1993). *Manual for the Beck Anxiety Inventory.* San Antonio, TX: Psychological Corporation.

Beck, A. T., Emery, G., & Greenberg, R. (1985). *Anxiety disorders and phobias: A cognitive perspective.* New York: Basic Books.

Beck, A. T., Rush, A. J., Shaw, B. F., & Emery, G. (1979). *Cognitive therapy of depression.* New York: Guilford Press.

Beck, A. T., Steer, R. A., & Brown, G. (1996). *Manual for the Beck Depression Inventory-II.* San Antonio, TX: Psychological Corporation.

Beck, J. S. (1995). *Cognitive therapy: Basics and beyond.* New York: Guilford Press.

Beidel, D. C., Christ, M. A., & Long, P. (1991). Somatic complaints in anxious children. *Journal of Abnormal Child Psychology, 19,* 659–670.

Beidel, D. C., & Turner, S. M. (1997). At risk for anxiety: I. Psychopathology in the offspring of anxious parents. *Journal of the American Academy of Child and Adolescent Psychiatry, 36,* 918–924.

Bell-Dolan, D. J., & Wessler, A. E. (1994). Attributional style of anxious children: Extensions from cognitive theory and research on adult anxiety. *Journal of Anxiety Disorders, 8,* 79–96.

Benson, H., & Stuart, E. (1992). *The wellness book: The comprehensive guide to maintaining health and treating stress-related illness.* Secaucus, NJ: Birch Lane Press.

Berg, I., & Jackson, A. (1985). Teenage school refusers grow up: A follow-up study of 168 subjects, ten years on average after inpatient treatment. *British Journal of Psychiatry, 147,* 366–370.

Berney, T., Klovin, I., Bhate, S. R., Gauside, R. F., Jeans, J., Kay, B., & Scarth, L. (1981). School phobia: A therapeutic trial with clomipramine and short-term outcome. *British Journal of Psychiatry, 138,* 110–118.

Bernstein, G. A., Borchardt, C. M., Perwein, A. R., Crosby, R. D., Kushner, M. G., Thuras, P. D., & Last, C. G. (2000). Imipramine plus cognitive-behavioral therapy in the treatment of school refusal. *Journal of the American Academy of Child and Adolescent Psychiatry, 39,* 276–283.

Bernstein, G. A., Borkovec, T. D., & Hazlett-Stevens, H. (2000). *New directions in progressive relaxation training: A guidebook for helping professionals.* Westport, CT: Praeger.

Bernstein, G. A., Garfinkel, B. D., & Borchardt, C. M. (1990). Comparative studies of pharmacotherapy for school refusal. *Journal of the American Academy of Child and Adolescent Psychiatry, 29,* 773–781.

Bernstein, G. A., Hektner, J. M., Borchardt, C. M., & McMillan, M. H. (2001). Treatment of school refusal: One-year follow-up. *Journal of the American Academy of Child and Adolescent Psychiatry, 40,* 206–213.

Bernstein, G. A., Massie, E. D., Thuras, P. D., Perwein, A. R., Borchardt, C. M., & Crosby, R. D. (1997). Somatic symptoms in anxious-depressed school refusers. *Journal of the American Academy of Child and Adolescent Psychiatry, 36,* 661–668.

Beutler, L. E. (1991). Selective treatment matching: Systematic eclectic psychotherapy. *Psychotherapy, 28,* 457–462.

Biederman, J., Faraone, S. V., Hirshfeld-Becker, D. R., Friedman, D., Robin, J.

A., & Rosenbaum, J. F. (2001). Patterns of psychopathology and dysfunction in high-risk children of parents with panic disorder and major depression. *American Journal of Psychiatry, 158,* 49–57.

Biederman, J., Rosenbaum, J. F., Chaloff, J., & Kagan, J. (1995). Behavioral inhibition as a risk factor of anxiety disorders. In J. S. March (Ed.), *Anxiety disorders in children and adolescents* (p. 61–81). New York: Guilford Press.

Bird, H. R., Canino, G., Rubio-Stipec, M., Gould, M. S., Ribera, J., Sesman, M., Woodbury, M., Huertas-Goldman, S., Pagan, A., Sanchez-Lacay, A., & Moscoso, M. (1988). Estimates of the prevalence of childhood maladjustment in a community survey in Puerto Rico: The use of combined measures. *Archives of General Psychiatry, 45,* 1120–1126.

Birmaher, B., Axelson, D. A., Monk, K., Kalas, C., Clark, D. B., Ehmann., M., Bridge, J., Jungeun, H., & Brent, D. A. (2003). Fluoxetine for the treatment of childhood anxiety disorders. *Journal of the American Academy of Child and Adolescent Psychiatry, 42,* 415–423.

Birmaher, B., Waterman, S., Ryan, N., Cully, M., Balach, L., Ingram, J., & Brodsky, M. (1994). Fluoxetine for childhood anxiety disorders. *Journal of the American Academy of Child and Adolescent Psychiatry, 33*(7), 993–999.

Bogels, S., & Zigterman, D. (2000). Dysfunctional cognitions in children with social phobia, separation anxiety disorder, and generalized anxiety disorder. *Journal of Abnormal Child Psychology, 28,* 205–211.

Borkovec, T. D, Hazlett-Stevens, H., & Diaz, M. L. (1999). The role of positive beliefs about worry in generalized anxiety disorder and its treatment. *Clinical Psychology and Psychotherapy, 6,* 126–138.

Borkovec, T. D., Robinson, E., Pruzinsky, T., & DePree, J. A. (1983). Preliminary exploration of worry: Some characteristics and processes. *Behaviour Research and Therapy, 21,* 9–16.

Borkovec, T. D., & Roemer, L. (1995). Perceived functions of worry among generalized anxiety disorder subjects: Distraction from more emotionally distressing topics? *Journal of Behavior Therapy and Experimental Psychiatry, 26,* 25–30.

Bowen, F., Vitaro, F., Kerr, M., & Pelletier, D. (1995). Childhood internalizing problems: Prediction from kindergarten, effect of maternal overprotectiveness, and sex differences. *Development and Psychopathology, 7,* 481–498.

Bowen, R. C., Offord, D. R., & Boyle, M. H. (1990). The prevalence of overanxious disorder and separation anxiety disorder: Results from the Ontario child health study. *Journal of the American Academy of Child and Adolescent Psychiatry, 29,* 753–758.

Bowlby, J. (1969). *Attachment and loss: Vol. 1. Attachment.* London: Penguin Books.

Bowlby, J. (1973). *Attachment and loss: Vol. 2. Separation anxiety and anger.* New York: Basic Books.

Bowlby, J. (1982). *Attachment and loss: Vol 1. Attachment* (2nd ed.). New York: Basic Books.

Brady, E., & Kendall, P. C. (1992). Comorbidity of anxiety and depression in children and adolescents. *Psychological Bulletin, 111,* 244–255.

Breier, A., Charney, D., & Heninger, G. (1986). Agoraphobia with panic attacks. *Archives of General Psychiatry, 43,* 1029–1036.

Brown, T. A., Chorpita, B. F., & Barlow, D. H. (1998). Structural relationships among dimensions of the DSM-IV anxiety and mood disorders and dimensions of negative affect, positive affect, and autonomic arousal. *Journal of Abnormal Psychology, 107,* 179–192.

Brynska, A., & Wolanczyk, T. (1998). Obsessive–compulsive disorder and separation anxiety. *Journal of the American Academy of Child and Adolescent Psychiatry, 37*(4), 350–351.

Buckley, M. E., Klein, D. N., Durbin, E. C., Hayden, E. P., & Moerk, K. C. (2002). Development and validation of a *q*-sort procedure to assess temperament and behavior in preschool age children. *Journal of Clinical Child and Adolescent Psychology, 31,* 525–539.

Burke, C. B., Burke, J. D., Regier, D. A., & Rae, D. S. (1990). Age at onset of selected mental disorders in five community populations. *Archives of General Psychiatry, 47,* 511–518.

Buss, A. H., & Plomin, R. (1984). *Temperament: Early developing personality traits.* Hillsdale, NJ: Erlbaum.

Calkins, S. D., & Fox, N. A. (1992). The relations among infant temperament, security of attachment, and behavioral inhibition at twenty-four months. *Child Development, 63,* 1456–1472.

Campbell, S. B. (1986). Developmental issues in childhood anxiety. In R. Gittelman (Ed.), *Anxiety disorders of childhood.* New York: Guilford Press.

Cantwell, D. P., & Baker, L. (1989). Stability and natural history of DSM-III childhood diagnoses. *Journal of the American Academy of Child and Adolescent Psychiatry, 28,* 691–700.

Cartwright-Hatton, S., & Wells, A. (1997). Beliefs about worry and intrusions: The Meta-Cognitions Questionnaire and its correlates. *Journal of Anxiety Disorders, 11,* 279–296.

Caspi, A., Henry, B., McGee, R. O., Moffitt, T., & Silva, P. A. (1995). Temperamental origins of child and adolescent behavior problems: From age three to age fifteen. *Child Development, 66,* 55–68.

Cassidy, J., & Berlin, L. J. (1994). The insecure/ambivalent pattern of attachment: Theory and research. *Child Development, 65,* 971–991.

Chess, S., & Thomas, A. (1984). *Origins and evolutions of behavior disorders.* New York: Brunner/Mazel.

Choate, M. L., & Pincus, D. B. (2001). *The Weekly Record of Anxiety at Separation (WRAS).* Unpublished assessment measure, Boston University, Center for Anxiety and Related Disorders.

Chorpita, B. F., Albano, A. M., & Barlow, D. H. (1996). Cognitive processing in children: Relationship to anxiety and family influences. *Journal of Clinical Child Psychology, 25,* 170–176.

Chorpita, B. F., Albano, A. M., & Barlow, D. H. (1998). The structure of negative emotions in a clinical sample of children and adolescents. *Journal of Abnormal Psychology, 107,* 74–85.

Chorpita, B. F., Brown, T. A., & Barlow, D. H. (1998). Perceived control as a mediator of family environment in etiological models of childhood anxiety. *Behavior Therapy, 29*, 457–476.

Chorpita, B. F., Taylor, A. A., Francis, S. E., Moffitt, C., & Austin, A. A. (2004). Efficacy of modular cognitive behavior therapy for childhood anxiety disorders. *Behavior Therapy, 35*, 263–287.

Cobham, V. E., Dadds, M. R., & Spence, S. H. (1998). The role of parental anxiety in the treatment of childhood anxiety. *Journal of Consulting and Clinical Psychology, 66*, 893–905.

Cobham, V. E., Dadds, M. R., & Spence, S. H. (1999). Anxious children and their parents: What do they expect? *Journal of Clinical Child Psychology, 28*, 220–231.

Cohen, P., Cohen, J., & Brook, J. (1993). An epidemiological study of disorders in late childhood and adolescence: II. Persistence of disorders. *Journal of Child Psychology and Psychiatry, 34*(6), 869–877.

Compton, S. N., Nelson, A. H., & March, J. S. (2000). Social phobia and separation anxiety symptoms in community and clinical samples of children and adolescents. *Journal of The American Academy of Child and Adolescent Psychiatry, 39*, 1040–1046.

Conners, C. K. (1997). *Conners Rating Scales–Revised*. North Tonawanda, NY: MultiHealth Systems.

Conners, C. K., & March, J. S. (1996). *Conners–March Developmental Questionnaire*. Toronto: MultiHealth Systems.

Costello, E. J., & Angold, A. (1995). Epidemiology. In J. S. March (Ed.), *Anxiety disorders in children and adolescents* (pp. 109–124). New York: Guilford Press.

Costello, A. J., Edelbrock, C. S., Dulcan, M. K., Kalas, R., & Klaric, S. H. (1984). *Report to NIMH on the NIMH Diagnostic Interview Schedule for Children (DISC)*. Washington, DC: National Institute of Mental Health.

Cowan, P. A., Cohn, D. A., Pape-Cowan, C. P., & Pearson, J. L. (1996). Parents' attachment histories and children's externalizing and internalizing behaviors. *Journal of Consulting and Clinical Psychology, 64*, 53–63.

Cox, C., Fedio, P., & Rapoport, J. (1989). Neuropsychological testing of obsessive–compulsive adolescents. In J. Rapoport (Ed.), *Obsessive–compulsive disorder in children and adolescents* (pp. 73–86). Washington DC: American Psychiatric Press.

Craske, M. G. (1999). *Anxiety disorders: Psychological approaches to theory and treatment*. Boulder, CO: Westview Press.

Dadds, M. R., Barrett, P. M., Rapee, R. M., & Ryan, S. M. (1996). Family process and child anxiety and aggression: An observational analysis. *Journal of Abnormal Child Psychology, 24*, 715–734.

Dadds, M. R., Holland, D. E., Spence, S. H., Laurens, K. R., Mullins, M., & Barrett, P. M. (1999). Early intervention and prevention of anxiety disorders in children: Results at 2-year follow-up. *Journal of Consulting and Clinical Psychology, 67*, 145–150.

DeWolff, M. S., & van Ijzendoorn, M. H. (1997). Sensitivity and attachment: A metanalysis on parental antecedents of infant attachment. *Child Development, 66*, 571–591.

Dumas, J. E., LaFreniere, P. J., & Serketich, W. J. (1995). Balance of power: A transactional analysis of control in mother–child dyads involving socially competent, aggressive, and anxious children. *Journal of Abnormal Psychology, 104,* 104–113.

D'Zurilla, T. J. (1986). *Problem-solving therapy: A social competence approach to clinical intervention.* New York: Springer.

Egger, H. L., Angold, A., & Costello, E. J. (1998). Headaches and psychopathology in children and adolescents. *Journal of the American Academy of Child and Adolescent Psychiatry, 37,* 951–958.

Egger, H. L., Costello, E. J., & Angold, A. (2003). School refusal and psychiatric disorders: A community study. *Journal of the American Academy of Child and Adolescent Psychiatry, 42,* 797–807.

Egger, H. L., Costello, E. J., Erkanli, A., & Angold, A. (1999). Somatic complaints and psychopathology in children and adolescents: Stomach aches, musculoskeletal pains, and headaches. *Journal of the American Academy of Child and Adolescent Psychiatry, 38,* 852–860.

Eisen, A. R., Engler, L. B., & Geyer, B. (1998). Parent training for separation anxiety disorder. In J. M. Briemeister & C. E. Schaefer (Eds.), *Handbook of parent training* (pp. 205–224). New York: Wiley.

Eisen, A. R., & Kearney, C. A. (1995). *Practitioner's guide to treating fear and anxiety in children and adolescents: A cognitive behavioral approach.* Northvale, NJ: Jason Aronson.

Eisen, A. R., Raleigh, H., & Neuhoff, C. (2003, November). *The unique impact of parent training for separation anxiety disorder.* Symposium conducted at the meeting of the Association for Advancement of Behavior Therapy, Boston.

Eisen, A. R., Rapee, R. M., & Barlow, D. H. (1990). The effects of breathing rate and pCO2 levels on relaxation and anxiety in a non-clinical population. *Journal of Anxiety Disorders, 4,* 183–190.

Eisen, A. R., & Silverman, W. K. (1993). Should I relax or change my thoughts?: A preliminary examination of cognitive therapy, relaxation training, and their combination with overanxious children. *Journal of Cognitive Psychotherapy: An International Quarterly, 7,* 265–279.

Eisen, A. R., & Silverman, W. K. (1998). Prescriptive treatment of generalized anxiety disorder in children. *Behavior Therapy, 29,* 105–121.

Eisen, A. R., Spasaro, S., Brien, L. K., Kearney, C. A., & Albano, A. M. (2004). Parental expectancies and childhood anxiety disorders: Psychometric properties of the parental expectancies scale. *Journal of Anxiety Disorders, 18,* 89–109.

Elkind, D. (2001). *The hurried child: Growing up too fast too soon.* Cambridge, MA: Perseus.

Emde, R. N., Gaensbauer, T. J., & Harmon, R. J. (1976). *Emotional expressions in infancy.* New York: International Universities Press.

Englund, M. M., Levy, A. K., Hyson, D. M., & Sroufe, L. A. (2000). Adolescent social competence: Effectiveness in a group setting. *Child Development, 71,* 1049–1060.

Epkins, C. C. (1996). Cognitive specificity and affective confounding in social anxiety and dysphoria in children. *Journal of Psychopathology and Behavioral Assessment, 18,* 83–101.

Farach, C. (2002). Separation anxiety disorder in a community sample of young adolescents. *Dissertation Abstracts International, 62*(7-B), 3133.

Fergusson, D. M., Horwood, D. J., & Lynskey, M. T. (1993). Prevalence and comorbidity of DSM-III-R diagnoses in a birth cohort of 15 year olds. *Journal of the American Academy of Child and Adolescent Psychiatry, 32,* 1127–1134.

Fischer, D. J., Himle, J. A., & Thyer, B. A. (1999). Separation anxiety disorder. In R. T. Ammerman, M. Hersen, & C. G. Last (Eds.), *Handbook of prescriptive treatments for children and adolescents* (pp. 141–154). Boston: Allyn & Bacon.

Fitzgibbons, L., & Pedrick, C. (2003). *Helping your child with OCD: A workbook for parents of children with obsessive–compulsive disorder.* Oakland, CA: New Harbinger.

Fonagy, P., Leigh, T., Steele, M., Steele, H., Kennedy, R., Mattoon, G., Target, M., & Gerber, A. (1996). The relation of attachment status, psychiatric classification, and response to psychotherapy. *Journal of Consulting and Clinical Psychology, 64,* 22–31.

Fox, N. A., & Calkins, S. D. (2003). The development of self-control of emotion: Intrinsic and extrinsic influences. *Motivation and Emotion, 27,* 7–26.

Frances, A., Widiger, T., & Fyer, M. R. (1990). The influence of classification methods on comorbidity. In J. D. Maser & C. R. Cloninger (Eds.), *Comorbidity of mood and anxiety disorders.* Washington, DC: American Psychiatric Press.

Francis, G., Last, C. G., & Strauss, C. C. (1987). Expression of separation anxiety disorder: The roles of gender and age. *Child Psychiatry and Human Development, 18,* 82–89.

Freedheim, D. K., & Shapiro, J. P. (1999). *The clinical child documentation sourcebook: A comprehensive collection of forms and guidelines for efficient record-keeping in child mental health practice.* New York: Wiley.

Friedberg, R. D. (1994). Storytelling and cognitive therapy with children. *Journal of Cognitive Therapy, 8,* 209–217.

Friedberg, R. D., Friedberg, B. A., & Friedberg, R. J. (2001). *Therapeutic exercises for children: Guided self-discovery through cognitive-behavioral techniques.* Sarasota, FL: Professional Resource Press.

Friedberg, R. D., & McClure, J. M. (2002). *Clinical practice of cognitive therapy with children and adolescents: The nuts and bolts.* New York: Guilford Press.

Fyer, A. J., Mannuzza, S., Chapman, T. F., Martin, L. Y., & Klein, D. F. (1995). Specificity in familial aggregation of phobic disorders. *Archives of General Psychiatry, 52,* 564–573.

Garland, E. J., & Smith, D. H. (1991). Simultaneous prepubertal onset of panic disorder, night terrors, and somnambulism. *Journal of the American Academy of Child and Adolescent Psychiatry, 30,* 553–555.

Geller, D., Biederman, J., Griffin, S., Jones, J., & Lefkowitz, T. (1996) Comorbidity of juvenile obsessive–compulsive disorder in children and adolescents: Phenomenology and family history. *Journal of the American Academy of Child and Adolescent Psychiatry, 35,* 1637–1646.

Ginsburg, G. S., & Schlossberg, M. C. (2002). Family-based treatment of child-hood anxiety disorders. *International Review of Psychiatry, 14*, 143–154.

Ginsburg, G. S., Silverman, W. K., & Kurtines, W. S. (1995). Cognitive-behavioral group therapy. In A. R., Eisen, C. A. Kearney, & C. E. Schaefer (Eds.), *Clinical handbook of anxiety disorders in children and adolescents.* Northvale, NJ: Jason Aronson.

Gittelman-Klein, R., & Klein, D. F. (1980). Separation anxiety in school refusal and its treatment with drugs. In L. Hersov & I Berg (Eds.), *Out of school: Modern perspectives on truancy and school refusal* (pp. 188–203). Chichester, UK: Wiley.

Goodwin, R., Lipsitz, J. D., Chapman, T. F., Manuzza, S., Fyer, A. J. (2001). Obsessive–compulsive disorder and separation anxiety comorbidity in early onset panic disorder. *Psychological Medicine, 31*(7), 1307–1310.

Graae, F., Milner, J., Rizzotto, L., & Klein, R. G. (1994). Clonazepam in child-hood anxiety disorders. *Journal of the American Academy of Child and Adolescent Psychiatry, 33*, 372–376.

Greenberg, M. T. (1999). Attachment and psychopathology in childhood. In J. Cassidy & P. R. Shaver (Eds.), *Handbook of attachment: Theory, research, and clinical applications* (pp. 469–496). New York: Guilford Press.

Greenham, S. L. (1999). Learning disabilities and psychosocial adjustment: A critical review. *Child Neuropsychology, 5*, 171–196.

Hahn, L., Hajinlian, J., Eisen, A. R., Winder, B., & Pincus, D. B. (2003, November). *Measuring the dimensions of separation anxiety and early panic in children and adolescents: The Separation Anxiety Assessment Scale.* Symposium conducted at the meeting of the Association for Advancement of Behavior Therapy, Boston.

Hajinlian, J., Hahn, L., Eisen, A. R., Zilli-Richardson, L., Reddy, R. A., Winder, B., & Pincus, D. B. (2003, November). *The phenomenon of separation anxiety across DSM-IV internalizing and externalizing disorders.* Paper presented at the meeting of the Association for Advancement of Behavior Therapy, Boston.

Hansburg, H. G. (1972). Separation problems of displaced children. In R. S. Parker (Ed.), *Emotional stress of war, violence, and peace.* Oxford, UK: Stanwix House.

Hayes, S. C., Barlow, D. H., & Nelson-Gray, R. O. (1999). *The scientist practitioner: Research and accountability in the age of managed care* (2nd ed.). Boston: Allyn & Bacon.

Hayward, C., Killen, J. D., Kraemer, H. C., & Taylor, C. B. (2000). Predictors of panic attacks in adolescents. *Journal of the American Academy of Child and Adolescent Psychiatry, 39*(2), 207–214.

Hayward, C., Killen, J. D., & Taylor, C. B. (1989). Panic attacks in young adolescents. *American Journal of Psychiatry, 146*, 1061–1062.

Hayward, C., Taylor, C. B., Blair-Greiner, A., & Strachowski, D. (1995). School refusal in young adolescent girls with nonclinical panic attacks. *Journal of Anxiety Disorders, 9*, 329–338.

Herjanic, B., & Reich, W. (1982). Development of a structured psychiatric interview for children: Agreement between child and parent on individual symptoms. *Journal of Abnormal Child Psychology, 10*, 307–324.

Hirshfeld, D. R., Biederman, J., Brody, L., & Faraone, S. V. (1997). Associations between expressed emotion and child behavioral inhibition and psychopathology: A pilot study. *Journal of the American Academy of Child and Adolescent Psychiatry, 36,* 205–213.

Hirshfeld, D. R., Rosenbaum, J. F., Biederman, J., Bolduc, E. A., Faraone, S. V., Snidman, N., Reznick, J. S., & Kagan, J. (1992). Stable behavioral inhibition and its association with anxiety disorder. *Journal of the American Academy of Child and Adolescent Psychiatry, 31,* 103–111.

Hodges, K., Kline, J., Stern, L., Cytryn, L., & McKnew, D. (1982). The development of a child assessment interview for research and clinical use. *Journal of Abnormal Child Psychology, 10,* 173–189.

House, A. E. (2002). *The first session with children and adolescents: Conducting a comprehensive mental health evaluation.* New York: Guilford Press.

Hudson, J. L., & Rapee, R. M. (2001). Parent–child interactions and anxiety disorders: An observational study. *Behaviour Research and Therapy, 39,* 1411–1427.

Ialongo, N., Edelsohn, G., Werthamer-Larsson, L., Crockett, L., & Kellam, S. (1994). The significance of self-reported anxious symptoms in first-grade children. *Journal of Abnormal Child Psychology, 22,* 441–455.

Isabella, R. A. (1993). Origins of attachment: Maternal interactive behavior across the first year. *Child Development, 64,* 605–621.

Isabella, R. A. (1994). The origins of infant–mother attachment: Maternal behavior and infant development. In R. Vasta (Ed.), *Annals of child development* (Vol. 10). London: Kingsley.

Izard, C. E. (1994). Innate and universal facial expressions: Evidence from developmental and cross-cultural research. *Psychological Bulletin, 115,* 288–299.

Jacobsen, E. (1974). *Progressive relaxation.* Chicago: University of Chicago Press.

Johnston, C., & Mash, E. J. (1989). A measure of parenting satisfaction and efficacy. *Journal of Clinical Child Psychology, 18,* 167–175.

Kaduson, H. G., & Schaefer, C. E. (1997). *101 favorite play therapy techniques.* Northvale, NJ: Jason Aronson.

Kaduson, H. G., & Schaefer, C. E. (2001). *101 more favorite play therapy techniques.* Northvale, NJ: Jason Aronson.

Kagan, J. (1989). Temperamental contributions to social behavior. *American Psychologist, 44,* 668–674.

Kagan, J. (1994). *Galen's prophecy.* New York: Basic Books.

Kagan, J. (1997). Temperament and the reactions to unfamiliarity. *Child Development, 68,* 139–143.

Kagan, J., Arcus, D., & Snidman, N. (1994). Reactivity in infants: A cross-national comparison. *Developmental Psychology, 30,* 342–345.

Kagan, J., Kearsley, R. B., & Zelazo, P. (1978). *Infancy: Its place in human development.* Cambridge, MA: Harvard University Press.

Kearney, C. A. (1993). Depression and school refusal behavior: A review with comments on classification and treatment. *Journal of School Psychology, 31,* 267–279.

Kearney, C. A. (2001). *School refusal behavior in youth: A functional approach to assessment and treatment.* Washington, DC: American Psychological Association.

Kearney, C. A., & Albano, A. M. (2000). *Therapist's guide to school refusal behavior.* San Antonio, TX: Psychological Corporation.

Kearney, C. A., & Albano, A. M. (2004). The functional profiles of school refusal behavior: Diagnostic aspects. *Behavior Modification, 28,* 147–161.

Kearney, C. A., Albano, A. M., Eisen, A. R., Allen, W. D., & Barlow, D. H. (1997). The phenomenology of panic disorder in youngsters: An empirical study of a clinical sample. *Journal of Anxiety Disorders, 11,* 49–62.

Kearney, C. A., & Silverman, W. K. (1990). A preliminary analysis of a functional model of assessment and treatment for school refusal behavior. *Behavior Modification, 14,* 340–366.

Kearney, C. A., & Silverman, W. K. (1992). Let's not push the "panic" button: A critical analysis of panic and panic disorder in adolescents. *Clinical Psychology Review, 12,* 293–305.

Kearney, C. A., & Silverman, W. K. (1995). Family environment of youngsters with school refusal behavior: A synopsis with implications for assessment and treatment. *The American Journal of Family Therapy, 23,* 59–72.

Kearney, C. A., & Silverman, W. K. (1996). The evolution and reconciliation of taxonomic strategies for school refusal behavior. *Clinical Psychology: Science and Practice, 3,* 339–354.

Kearney, C. A., & Silverman, W. K. (1999). Functionally-based prescriptive and nonprescriptive treatment for children and adolescents with school refusal behavior. *Behavior Therapy, 30,* 673–695.

Kearney, C. A., Silverman, W. K., & Eisen, A. R. (1989, October). *Characteristics of children and adolescents with school refusal behavior.* Paper presented at the meeting of the Berkshire Conference of Behavior Analysis and Therapy, Amherst, MA.

Kendall, P. C. (1990). *The coping cat workbook.* Philadelphia: Temple University, Department of Psychology.

Kendall, P. C. (1992). Healthy thinking. *Behavior Therapy, 23,* 1–11.

Kendall, P. C. (1994). Treating anxiety disorders in children: Results of a randomized clinical trial. *Journal of Consulting and Clinical Psychology, 62*(1), 100–110.

Kendall, P. C. (2000). Guiding theory for therapy with children and adolescents. In P. C. Kendall (Ed.), *Child and adolescent therapy: Cognitive-behavioral procedures* (2nd ed., pp. 3–27). New York: Guilford Press.

Kendall, P. C., Brady, E. U., & Verduin, T. L. (2001). Comorbidity in childhood anxiety disorders and treatment outcome. *Journal of the American Academy of Child and Adolescent Psychiatry, 40,* 787–794.

Kendall, P. C., & Chansky, T. E. (1991). Considering cognition in anxiety-disordered children. *Journal of Anxiety Disorders, 5,* 167–185.

Kendall, P. C., Chansky, T. E., Kane, M. T., Kim, R. S., Kortlander, E., Ronan, K. R., Sessa, F. M., & Siqueland, L. (1992). *Anxiety disorders in youth: Cognitive-behavioral interventions.* Boston: Allyn & Bacon.

Kendall, P. C., Flannery-Schroeder, E., Panichelli-Mindel, S. M., Southam-Gerow, M., Henin, A., & Warman, M. (1997). Therapy for youths with anxiety disorders: A second randomized clinical trial. *Journal of Consulting and Clinical Psychology, 65*(3), 366–380.

Kendall, P. C., Safford, S., Flannery-Schroeder, E., & Webb, A. (2004). Child anxiety treatment outcomes in adolescence and impact on substance abuse and depression at 7.4-year follow-up. *Journal of Consulting and Clinical Psychology, 72*, 276–287.

Klagsbrun, M., & Bowlby, J. (1976). Responses to separation from parents: A clinical test for young children. *British Journal of Projective Psychology and Personality Study, 21*, 7–27.

Klein, D. F., Zitrin, C. M., Woerner, M. G., & Ross, D. C. (1983). Treatment of phobias: II. Behavior therapy and supportive psychotherapy: Are there any specific ingredients? *Archives of General Psychiatry, 40*, 139–145.

Klein, R. G., Koplewicz, H. S., & Kanner, A. (1992). Imipramine treatment of children with separation anxiety disorder. *Journal of the American Academy of Child and Adolescent Psychiatry, 31*, 21–28.

Knell, S. M. (1993). *Cognitive-behavior play therapy.* Northvale, NJ: Jason Aronson.

Knox, L. S., Albano, A. M., & Barlow, D. H. (1996). Parental involvement in the treatment of childhood obsessive–compulsive disorder: A multiple-baseline examination incorporating parents. *Behavior Therapy, 27*, 93–114.

Kochanska, G. (1998). Mother–child relationships, child fearfulness, and emerging attachment: A short-term longitudinal study. *Developmental Psychology, 34*, 480–490.

Kochanska, G. (2001). Emotional development in children with different attachment histories: The first three years. *Child Development, 72*, 474–490.

Kortlander, E., Kendall, P. C., & Panichelli-Mindell, S. M. (1997). Maternal expectations and attributions about coping in anxious children. *Journal of Anxiety Disorders, 11*, 297–315.

Kovacs, M. (1992). *Children's Depression Inventory manual.* North Tonawanda, NY: MultiHealth Systems.

Laraia, M. T., Stuart, G. W., Frye, L. H., Lydiard, R. B., & Ballenger, J. C. (1994). Childhood environment of women having panic disorder with agoraphobia. *Journal of Anxiety Disorders, 8*, 1–17.

Last, C. G. (1991). Somatic complaints in anxiety disordered children. *Journal of Anxiety Disorders, 5*, 125–138.

Last, C. G., Francis, G., & Strauss, C. C. (1989). Assessing fears in anxiety-disordered children with the revised Fear Survey Schedule for Children (FSSC-R). *Journal of Clinical Child Psychology, 18*, 137–141.

Last, C. G., Hersen, M., Kazdin, A. E., Finkelstein, R., & Strauss, C. C. (1987). Comparison of DSM-III separation anxiety and overanxious disorders: Demographic characteristics and patterns of comorbidity. *Journal of the American Academy of Child Psychiatry, 26*, 527–531.

Last, C. G., Perrin, S., Hersen, M., & Kazdin, A. (1996). A prospective study of childhood anxiety disorders. *Journal of the American Academy of Child and Adolescent Psychiatry, 35*, 1502–1510.

Last, C. G., Perrin, S., Hersen, M., & Kazdin, A. E. (1992). DSM-III-R anxiety disorders in children: Socio-demographic and clinical characteristics. *Journal of the American Academy of Child and Adolescent Psychiatry, 31*, 1070–1076.

Last, C. G., Philips, J. E., & Statfield, A. (1987). Childhood anxiety disorders in mothers and their children. *Child Psychiatry and Human Development, 18*, 103–112.

Last, C. G., & Strauss, C. (1990). School refusal in anxiety-disordered children and adolescents. *Journal of the American Academy of Child and Adolescent Psychiatry, 29*, 31–35.

Last, C. G., Strauss, C., & Francis, G. (1987). Comorbidity among childhood anxiety disorders. *Journal of Nervous and Mental Disease, 175*(12), 726–730.

Leitenberg, H., Yost, L. W., & Carroll-Wilson, M. (1986). Negative cognitive errors in children: Questionnaire development, normative data, and comparisons between children with and without self-reported symptoms of depression, low self-esteem, and evaluation anxiety. *Journal of Consulting and Clinical Psychology, 54*, 528–536.

Leung, P., & Wong, M. (1998). Can cognitive distortions differentiate between internalizing and externalizing problems? *Journal of Clinical Child Psychology and Psychiatry and Allied Disciplines, 39*, 263–269.

Lipsitz, J. D., Martin, L. Y., Mannuzza, S., Chapman, T. F., Liebowitz, M. R., & Klein, D. F. (1994). Childhood separation anxiety disorder in patients with adult anxiety disorders. *American Journal of Psychiatry, 151*, 927–929.

Lonigan, C. J., & Philips, B. M. (2001). Temperamental basis of anxiety disorders in children. In M. W. Vasey & M. R. Dadds (Eds.), *The developmental psychopathology of anxiety* (pp. 60–91). New York: Oxford University Press.

Lonigan, C. J., Vasey, M. W., Philips, B. M., & Hazen, R. A. (2004). Temperament, anxiety, and the processing of threat-relevant stimuli. *Journal of Clinical Child and Adolescent Psychology, 33*, 8–20.

Lyness, D. (1993). Mastery of childhood fears. In C. E. Schaefer (Ed.), *The therapeutic powers of play* (pp. 309–322). Northvale, NJ: Jason Aronson.

Lyon, G. R. (1996). Learning disabilities. In E. J. Mash & R. A. Barkley (Eds.), *Child psychopathology* (pp. 390–435). New York: Guilford Press.

Lytton, H. (1990). Child and parent effects in boys' conduct disorder: A reinterpretation. *Developmental Psychology, 26*, 683–697.

Main, M., Kaplan, N., & Cassidy, J. (1985). Security in infancy, childhood, and adulthood: A move to the level of representation. *Monographs of the Society for Research in Child Development, 50*, 66–104.

Manicavasagar, V., Silove, D., & Curtis, J. (1997). Separation anxiety in adulthood: A phenomenological investigation. *Comprehensive Psychiatry, 38*, 274–282.

Manicavasagar, V., Silove, D., Curtis, J., & Wagner, R. (2000). Continuities of separation anxiety from early life to adulthood: A clinic study. *Journal of Anxiety Disorders, 14*, 1–18.

Manicavasagar, V., Silove, D., Rapee, R., Waters, F., & Momartin, S. (2001). Parent–child concordance for separation anxiety: A clinical study. *Journal of Affective Disorders, 65*, 81–84.

March, J. S. (1997). *Multidimensional Anxiety Scale for Children*. North Tonawanda, NY: MultiHealth Systems.

March, J. S. (2002). Combining medication and psychosocial treatments: An evidence-based medicine approach. *International Review of Psychiatry, 14*, 155–163.

March, J. S., & Mulle, K. (1998). *OCD in children and adolescents: A cognitive-behavioral treatment manual*. New York: Guilford Press.

Marks, I. M. (1987). *Fears, phobias, and rituals: Panic, anxiety, and their disorders*. New York: Oxford University Press.

Marks, I. M., & Mathews, A. M. (1979). Brief standard self-rating for phobic patients. *Behaviour Research and Therapy, 17*, 263–267.

Marlatt, G. A. (1985). Relapse prevention: Theoretical rationale and overview of the model. In G. A. Marlatt & J. R. Gordon (Eds.), *Relapse prevention: Maintenance strategies in the treatment of addictive behaviors* (pp. 3–70). New York: Guilford Press.

Martin, G., & Pear, J. (1983). *Behavior modification: What it is and how to do it* (2nd ed.). New York: Pergamon Press.

Masi, G., Favilla, L., Mucci, M., & Millepiedi, S. (2000). Panic disorder in clinically referred children and adolescents. *Child Psychiatry and Human Development, 31*, 139–151.

Masi, G., Mucci, M., Favilla, L., Romano, R., & Poli, P. (1999). Symptomatology and comorbidity of generalized anxiety disorder in children and adolescents. *Comprehensive Psychiatry, 40*, 210–215.

Masi, G., Mucci, M., & Millepiedi, S. (2001). Separation anxiety disorder in children and adolescents: Epidemiology, diagnosis and management. *CNS Drugs, 15*, 93–104.

Mattis, S. G., & Ollendick, T. H. (1997). Panic in children and adolescents: A developmental analysis. In T. H. Ollendick & R. J. Prinz (Eds.), *Advances in Clinical Child Psychology, 19* (pp. 27–74). New York: Plenum Press.

Mattis, S. G., & Pincus, D. B. (2004). Treatment of SAD and panic disorder in children and adolescents. In P. M. Barrett & T. H. Ollendick (Eds.), *Handbook of interventions that work with children and adolescents: Prevention and treatment* (pp. 145–168). New York: Wiley.

Maziade, M., Caron, C., Cote, R., Merette, C., Bernier, H., LaPlante, B., Boutin, P., & Thivierge, J. (1990). Psychiatric status of adolescents who had extreme temperaments at age 7. *American Journal of Psychiatry, 147*, 1531–1536.

McClure, E. B., Brennan, P. A., Hammen, C., & LeBrocque, R. M. (2001). Parental anxiety disorders, child anxiety disorders, and the perceived parent–child relationship in an Australian high-risk sample. *Journal of Abnormal Child Psychology, 29*, 1–10.

McGee, R., Feehan, M., Williams, S., & Anderson, J. (1992). DSM-III disorders from age 11 to age 15 years. *Journal of the American Academy of Child and Adolescent Psychiatry, 31*, 50–59.

McKinney, W. T. (1985). Separation and depression: Biological markers. In M. Reite & T. Field (Eds.), *The psychobiology of attachment* (pp. 201–222). New York: Wiley.

McMahon, R. J., & Forehand, R. L. (2003). *Helping the noncompliant child: Family-based treatment for oppositional behavior* (2nd ed.). New York: Guilford Press.

McNally, R. J., & Eke, M. (1996). Anxiety, sensitivity, suffocation fear, and breath-holding duration as predictors of response to carbon dioxide challenge. *Journal of Abnormal Psychology, 105,* 146–149.

Menzies, R. G., & Harris, L. M. (2001). Nonassociative factors in the development of phobias. In M. W. Vasey & M. R. Dadds (Eds.), *The developmental psychopathology of anxiety* (pp. 183–230). New York: Oxford University Press.

Millon, T., Millon, C., & Davis, R. (1994). *Millon Clinical Multiaxial Inventory–III.* Minneapolis, MN: National Computer Systems.

Mineka, S. (1982). Depression and helplessness in primates. In H. E. Fitzgerald, J. A. Mullins, & P. Gaze (Eds.), *Child nurturance* (Vol. 3, pp. 197–242). New York: Plenum Press.

Moos, R. H., & Moos, B. S. (1986). *Family Environment Scale manual* (2nd ed.). Palo Alto, CA: Consulting Psychologists Press.

Muris, P., Meesters, C., Merckelbach, H., Sermon, A., & Zwakhalen, S. (1998). Worry in normal children. *Journal of the American Academy of Child and Adolescent Psychiatry, 37,* 703–710.

Muris, P., Merckelbach, H., Gadet, B., & Moulaert, V. (2000). Fears, worries, and scary dreams in 4 to 12 year-old children: Their content, developmental pattern, and origins. *Journal of Clinical Child Psychology, 29,* 43–52.

Muris, P., Merckelbach, H., Meesters, C., & van den Brand, K. (2002). Cognitive development and worry in normal children. *Cognitive Therapy and Research, 26,* 775–787.

Nelles, W. B., & Barlow, D. H. (1988). Do children panic? *Clinical Psychology Review, 8,* 359–372.

Neuhoff, C., Hahn, L., & Eisen, A. R. (November, 2003). *The prescriptive treatment of separation anxiety disorder: CBT versus parent training.* Symposium conducted at the meeting of the Association for Advancement of Behavior Therapy, Boston.

Ollendick, T. H. (1983). Reliability and validity of the revised Fear Survey Schedule for Children (FSSC-R). *Behaviour Research and Therapy, 21,* 685–692.

Ollendick, T. H. (1998). Panic disorder in children and adolescents: New developments, new directions. *Journal of Clinical Child Psychology, 27,* 234–245.

Ollendick, T. H., & Cerny, J. A. (1981). *Clinical behavior therapy with children.* New York: Kluwer/Plenum Press.

Ollendick, T. H., & King, N. J. (2002). Empirically supported treatments for children and adolescents. *International Review of Psychiatry, 14,* 387–424.

Ollendick, T. H., Lease, C. A., & Cooper, C. (1993). Separation anxiety in young adults: A preliminary examination. *Journal of Anxiety Disorders, 7,* 293–305.

Olsen, D. H., McCubbin, H. I., Barnes, H., et al. (1985). *Family inventories.* St. Paul, MN: Family Social Science.

Papp, L. A., Klein, D. F., & Gorman, J. M. (1993). Carbon dioxide hypersensitivity, hyperventilation, and panic disorder. *American Journal of Psychiatry,* *150,* 1149–1157.

Parker, G. (1990). The parental bonding instrument: A decade of research. *Psychiatry and Psychiatric Epidemiology, 25,* 281–282.

Pederson, D. R., & Moran, G. (1996). Expressions of the attachment relationship outside of the Strange Situation. *Child Development, 67,* 915–929.

Perna, G., Bertani, A., Arancio, C., Ronchi, & Bellodi, L. (1995). Laboratory response of patients with panic and obsessive–compulsive disorders to 35% CO2 challenges. *American Journal of Psychiatry, 152,* 85–89.

Perna, G., Bertani, A., Politi, E., Columbo, G., & Bellodi, L. (1997). Asthma and panic attacks. *Biological Psychiatry, 42,* 625–630.

Perrin, S., & Last, C. G. (1997). Worrisome thoughts in children clinically referred for anxiety disorder. *Journal of Clinical Child Psychology, 26,* 181–189.

Petti, V., Voelker, S., Shore, D. L., & Hayman-Abello, S. E. (2003). Perception of nonverbal emotion cues by children with nonverbal learning disabilities. *Journal of Developmental and Physical Disabilities, 15,* 23–36.

Piacentini, J., & Bergman, R. L. (2001). Developmental issues in cognitive therapy for childhood anxiety disorders. *Journal of Cognitive Psychotherapy: An International Quarterly, 15,* 165–182.

Piaget, J. (1967). *The child's conception of the world.* Totowa, NJ: Littlefield, Adams.

Piaget, J. (1970). Piaget's theory. In P. H. Mussen (Ed.), *Carmichaels's manual of child psychology* (Vol. 1, pp. 703–732). New York: Wiley.

Pilkington, C. L., & Piersel, W. C. (1991). School phobia: A critical analysis of the separation anxiety theory and an alternative explanation. *Psychology in the Schools, 28,* 290–303.

Pine, D. S. (2002). Development of the symptom of anxiety. In M. Lewis (Ed.), *Child and adolescent psychiatry* (3rd ed., pp. 343–351). Philadelphia: Lippincot, Williams & Wilkins.

Pine, D. S., Cohen, P., Gurley, D., Brook, J., & Ma, Y. (1998). The risk for early adulthood anxiety and depressive disorders in adolescents with anxiety and depressive disorders. *Archives of General Psychiatry, 55,* 56–64.

Pine, D. S., Klein, R. G., Coplan, J. D., Papp, L. A., Hoven, C. W., Martinez, J., Kovalenko, P., Mandell, D. J., Moreau, D., Klein, D. F., & Gorman, J. M. (2000). Differential carbon dioxide sensitivity in childhood anxiety disorders and non-ill comparison group. *Archives of General Psychiatry, 57,* 960–967.

Plomin, R., & Rowe, D. C. (1979). Genetic and environmental etiology of social behavior in infancy. *Developmental Psychology, 15,* 62–72.

Puig-Antich, J., Orvaschel, H., Tabrizi, M. A., & Chambers, W. J., (1980). *Schedule for Affective Disorders and Schizophrenia for school-aged children–epidemiologic version* (Kiddie-SADS-E; 3rd ed.). New York: New York State Psychiatric Institute.

Rabian, B., Peterson, R. A., Richters, J., & Jensen, P. S. (1993). Anxiety sensitivity among anxious children. *Journal of Clinical Child Psychology, 22,* 441–446.

Raleigh, H., Brien, L. K., & Eisen, A. R. (2001). *Parent training manual for separation anxious youth.* Teaneck, NJ: Fairleigh Dickinson University, School of Psychology.

Rapee, R. M. (1997). Potential role of childrearing practices in the development of anxiety and depression. *Clinical Psychology Review, 17,* 47–67.

Rapee, R. M. (2002). The development and modification of temperamental risk for anxiety disorders: Prevention of a lifetime of anxiety? *Biological Psychiatry, 52,* 947–957.

Rapee, R. M., Barrett, P. M., Dadds, M. R., & Evans, L. (1994). Reliability of the DSM-III-R anxiety disorders using structured interview: Interrater and parent–child agreement. *Journal of the American Academy of Child and Adolescent Psychiatry, 33,* 984–992.

Reich, W. (2000). Diagnostic Interview for Children and Adolescents (DICA). *Journal of the American Academy of Child and Adolescent Psychiatry, 39,* 59–66.

Reiss, S., Silverman, W. K., & Weems, C. F. (2001). Anxiety sensitivity. In M. W. Vasey & M. R. Dadds (Eds.), *The developmental psychopathology of anxiety* (pp. 92–111). New York: Oxford University Press.

Reynolds, C. R., & Richman, B. O. (1978). What I think and feel? A revised measure of children's manifest anxiety. *Journal of Abnormal Child Psychology, 6,* 271–280.

Reynolds, W. M. (1989). *Reynold's Child Depression Scale.* Odessa, FL: Psychological Assessment Resources.

Rietveld, S., Prins, P. J. M., & van Beest, I. (2002). Negative thoughts in children with symptoms of anxiety and depression. *Journal of Psychopathology and Behavioral Assessment, 24,* 107–113.

Rosen, B. C. (1998). *Winners and losers of the information revolution: Psychosocial change and its discontents.* Wesport, CT: Praeger.

Rosenbaum, J. F., Biederman, J., Hirshfeld, D. R., Bolduc, E. A., & Chaloff, J. (1991). Behavioral inhibition in children: A possible precursor to panic disorder and social phobia. *Journal of Clinical Psychiatry, 52,* 5–9.

Rosenstein, D. S., & Horowitz, H. A. (1996). Adolescent attachment and psychopathology. *Journal of Consulting and Clinical Psychology, 64,* 244–253.

Rourke, B. P. (Ed.). (1995). *Syndrome of nonverbal learning disabilities: Neurodevelopmental manifestations.* New York: Guilford Press.

Rubin, K. H., & Mills, R. S. L. (1991). Conceptualizing developmental pathways to internalizing disorders in childhood. *Canadian Journal of Behavioural Science, 23,* 300–317.

RUPP (Research Units of Psychopharmacology). (2001). Fluvoxamine for the treatment of anxiety disorders in children and adolescents. *New England Journal of Medicine, 344,* 1279–1285.

Rutter, M. (1981). *Scientific foundations of developmental psychiatry.* Baltimore: University Park Press.

Sackett, D., Richardson, W., Rosenberg, W. A., & Haynes, B. (2000). *Evidenced-based medicine* (2nd ed.). London: Churchill Livingston.

Schaefer, C. E., & Greenberg, R. (1997). Measurement of playfulness: A neglected therapist variable. *International Journal of Play Therapy, 6,* 21–31.

Schaefer, C. E., & Petronko, M. R. (1987). *Teach your baby to sleep through the night*. New York: Putnam.

Seifer, R., Schiller, M., Sameroff, A. J., Resnick, S., & Riordan, K. (1996). Attachment, maternal sensitivity, and infant temperament during the first year of life. *Developmental Psychology, 32,* 12–25.

Shaffer, D. R. (2002). *Developmental psychology* (6th ed.). Belmont, CA: Wadsworth/Thomson Learning.

Shaffer, D. R., Fisher, P., Lucas, C. P., Dulcan, M. K., & Schwab-Stone, M. E. (2000). NIMH Diagnostic Interview Schedule for Children—Version IV: Description, differences from previous versions, and reliability of some common diagnoses. *Journal of the American Academy of Child and Adolescent Psychiatry, 39,* 28–38.

Shiller, V. M., Izard, C. E., & Hembree, E. A. (1986). Patterns of emotion expression during separation in the Strange-Situation procedure. *Developmental Psychology, 22,* 378–382.

Shortt, A. L., Barrett, P. M., & Fox, T. L. (2001). Evaluating the FRIENDS program: A cognitive-behavioral group treatment for anxious children and their parents. *Journal of Clinical Child Psychology, 30,* 525–535.

Shouldice, A., & Stevenson-Hinde, J. (1992). Coping with security distress: The separation anxiety test and attachment classification at 4. 5 years. *Journal of Child Psychology and Psychiatry, 33,* 331–348.

Silove, D., Harris, M., Morgan, A., Boyce, P., Manicavasagar, V., Hadzi-Pavlovic, D., & Wilhelm, K. (1995). Is early separation anxiety a specific precursor of panic disorder-agoraphobia? A community study. *Psychological Medicine, 25,* 405–411.

Silove, D., & Manicavasagar, V. (1993). Adults who feared school: Is early separation anxiety specific to the pathogenesis of panic disorder? *Acta Psychiatrica Scandinavica, 88,* 385–390.

Silove, D., Manicavasagar, V., O'Connell, D., Blaszczyski, A., Wagner, R., & Henry, J. (1993). The development of the Separation Anxiety Symptom Inventory (SASI). *Australian New Zealand Journal of Psychiatry, 27,* 477–488.

Silverman, W. K. (1989). *Self-control manual for phobic children*. Unpublished treatment protocol, Florida International University, Department of Psychology.

Silverman, W. K. (1991). Diagnostic reliability of anxiety disorders in children using structured interviews. *Journal of Anxiety Disorders, 5,* 105–124.

Silverman, W. K., & Albano, A. M. (1996). *The Anxiety Disorders Interview Schedule for DSM-IV: Child and parent versions*. San Antonio, TX: Psychological Corporation.

Silverman, W. K., & Eisen, A. R. (1992). Age differences in the reliability of parent and child reports of child anxious symptomatology using a structured interview. *Journal of the American Academy of Child and Adolescent Psychiatry, 31,* 117–124.

Silverman, W. K., Fleisig, W., Rabian, B., & Peterson, R. A. (1991). The child anxiety sensitivity index. *Journal of Clinical Child Psychology, 20,* 162–168.

Silverman, W. K., & Kurtines, W. M. (1996a). *Anxiety and phobic disorders: A pragmatic approach.* New York: Plenum Press.

Silverman, W. K., & Kurtines, W. M. (1996b). Transfer of control: A psychosocial intervention model for internalizing disorders in youth. In E. D. Hibbs & P. S. Jensen (Eds.), *Psychosocial treatments for child and adolescent disorders: Empirically based strategies for clinical practice* (pp. 63–81). Washington, DC: American Psychological Association.

Silverman, W. K., La Greca, A. M., & Wassertein, S. (1995). What do children worry about?: Worries and their relation to anxiety. *Child Development, 66,* 671–686.

Silverman, W. K., & Nelles, W. B. (1988). The Anxiety Disorders Interview Schedule for children. *Journal of the American Academy of Child and Adolescent Psychiatry, 27,* 772–778.

Silverman, W. K., Saavedra, L. M., & Pina, A. A. (2001). Test–retest reliability of anxiety symptoms and diagnoses using the Anxiety Disorders Interview Schedule for DSM-IV: Child and parent versions. *Journal of the American Academy of Child and Adolescent Psychiatry, 40,* 937–944.

Simeon, J. G., Ferguson, H. B., Knott, V., Roberts, N., Gauthier, B., Dubois, C., & Wiggins, D. (1992). Clinical, cognitive, and neurophysiological effects of alprazolam in children and adolescents with overanxious and avoidant disorders. *Journal of the American Academy of Child and Adolescent Psychiatry, 31,* 29–33.

Simeon, J. G., Knott, V. J., Dubois, C., Wiggins, D., Geraets, I., Thatte, S., & Miller, W. (1994). Buspirone therapy of mixed anxiety disorders in childhood and adolescence: A pilot study. *Journal of Child and Adolescent Psychopharmacology, 4,* 159–170.

Simeon, J. G., & Wiggins, D. M. (1995). Pharmacotherapy. In A. R. Eisen, C. A. Kearney, & C. E. Schaefer (Eds.), *Clinical handbook of anxiety disorders in children and adolescents* (pp. 550–570). Northvale, NJ: Jason Aronson.

Siqueland, L., Kendall, P. C., & Steinberg, L. (1996). Anxiety in children: Perceived family environments and observed family interaction. *Journal of Clinical Child Psychology, 25,* 225–237.

Sloan, T. (1996). *Damaged life: The crisis of the modern psyche.* New York: Routledge.

Sorenson, L. G., Forbes, P., Bernstein, J. H., Weiler, M. D., Mitchell, W. M., & Waber, D. P. (2003). Psychosocial adjustment over a two-year period in children referred for learning problems: Risk, resilience, and adaptation. *Learning Disabilities Research and Practice, 18,* 10–24.

Southam-Gerow, M. A., Weisz, J. R., & Kendall, P. C. (2003). Youth with anxiety disorders in research and service clinics: Examining client differences and similarities. *Journal of Clinical Child and Adolescent Psychology, 32,* 375–385.

Spence, S. H. (1997). Structure of anxiety symptoms among children: A confirmatory factor–analytic study. *Journal of Abnormal Psychology, 106*(2), 280–297.

Spence, S. H. (2001). Prevention strategies. In M. W. Vasey & M. R. Dadds

(Eds.), *The developmental psychopathology of anxiety* (pp. 325–351). New York: Oxford University Press.

Spielberger, C. D. (1973). *Manual for the State–Trait Anxiety Inventory for Children*. Palo Alto, CA: Consulting Psychologists Press.

Spielberger, C. D., & Rickman, R. L. (1990). Assessment of state and trait anxiety. In N. Sartorius, V. Andreoli, G. Cassano, L. Eisenberg, P. Kielkolt, P. Pancheri, & G. Racagni (Eds.), *Anxiety: Psychobiological and clinical perspectives* (pp. 69–83). New York: Hemisphere.

Sroufe, L. A. (1990). Considering normal and abnormal together: The essence of developmental psychopathology. *Development and Psychopathology, 2*, 335–347.

Stark, K. D., Humphrey, L. L., Crook, K., & Lewis, K. (1990). Perceived family environments of depressed and anxious children. *Journal of Abnormal Child Psychology, 18*, 527–548.

Stewart, K. (2002). *Helping a child with a nonverbal learning disorder or Asperger's syndrome: A parent's guide*. Oakland, CA: New Harbinger.

Stickney, M. I., & Miltenberger, R. G. (1998). School refusal behavior: Prevalence, characteristics, and the schools' response. *Education and Treatment of Children, 21*, 160–170.

Tanguay, P. B. (2001). *Nonverbal learning disabilities at home: A parent's guide*. London: Kingsley.

Thomas, A., & Chess, S. (1977). *Temperament and development*. New York: Brunner/Mazel.

Thomas, A., & Chess, S. (1986). The New York longitudinal study: From infancy to early adult life. In R. Plomin & J. Dunn (Eds.), *The study of temperament: Changes, continuities, and challenges*. Hillsdale, NJ: Erlbaum.

Thomas, A., Chess, S., & Korn, S. (1982). The reality of difficult temperament. *Merrill–Palmer Quarterly, 28*, 1–20.

Thomasgard, M., & Metz, P. W. (1993). Parental overprotection revisited. *Child Psychiatry and Human Development, 24*, 67–80.

Thomasgard, M., Metz, P. W., Edelbrock, C., & Shonkoff, J. P. (1995). Parent-child relationship disorders: I. Parental overprotection and the development of the parent protection scale. *Journal of Developmental and Behavioral Pediatrics, 16*, 244–250.

Thompson, R. A., & Calkins, S. D. (1996). The double-edged sword: Emotional regulation for children at risk. *Development and Psychopathology, 8*, 163–182.

Thompson, R. A., & Limber, S. (1990). "Social anxiety" in infancy: Stranger wariness and separation distress. In H. Leitenberg (Ed.), *Handbook of social and evaluation anxiety* (pp. 85–137). New York: Plenum Press.

Thurber, C. A. (1995). The experience and expression of homesickness in preadolescent and adolescent boys. *Child Development, 66*, 1162–1178.

Thurber, C. A., Sigman, M. D., Weisz, J. R., & Schmidt, C. K. (1999). Homesickness in preadolescent girls: Risk factors, behavioral correlates, and sequelae. *Journal of Clinical Child Psychology, 28*, 185–196.

Thyer, B. A., Neese, R., Curtis, G., & Cameron, O. (1986). Panic disorder: A test of the separation anxiety hypothesis. *Behaviour Research and Therapy*, *24*, 209–211.

Treadwell, K. H., & Kendall, P. C. (1996). Self-talk in youth with anxiety disorders: States of mind, content specificity, and treatment outcome. *Journal of Consulting and Clinical Psychology*, *64*, 941–950.

Twenge, J. T. (2000). The age of anxiety?: Birth cohort change in anxiety and neuroticism, 1952–1993. *Journal of Personality and Social Psychology*, *79*, 1007–1021.

Valleni-Basile, L., Garrison, C., Jackson, K., Waller, J., McKeown, R., Addy, C., & Cuffe, S. (1994). Frequency of obsessive–compulsive disorder in a community sample of young adolescents. *Journal of the American Academy of Child and Adolescent Psychiatry*, *33* (6), 782–791.

van den Boom, D. C. (1994). The influence of temperament and mothering on attachment and exploration: An experimental manipulation of sensitive responsiveness among lower class mothers with irritable infants. *Child Development*, *65*, 1457–1477.

van derMolen, G., van der Hout, M., van Dieren, A., & Griez, E. (1989). Childhood separation anxiety and adult onset panic disorders. *Journal of Anxiety Disorders*, *3*, 97–106.

Vasey, M. W., Crnic, K. A., & Carter, W. G. (1994). Worry in childhood: A developmental perspective. *Cognitive Therapy and Research*, *18*, 529–549.

Vasey, M. W., & MacLeod, C. (2001). Information-processing factors in childhood anxiety: A review and developmental perspective. In M. W. Vasey & M. R. Dadds (Eds.), *The developmental psychopathology of anxiety* (pp. 253–277). New York: Oxford University Press.

Velosa, J. F., & Riddle, M. A. (2000). Pharmacologic treatment of anxiety disorders in children and adolescents. *Child and Adolescent Psychiatric Clinics of North America*, *9*, 119–133.

Verburg, K., Griez, E., Meijer, J., & Pols, H. (1995). Respiratory disorders as a possible predisposing factor for panic disorder. *Journal of Affective Disorders*, *33*, 129–134.

Verduin, T. L., & Kendall, P. C. (2003). Differential occurrence of comorbidity within childhood anxiety disorders. *Journal of Clinical Child and Adolescent Psychology*, *32*, 290–295.

Vitiello, B., Behar, D., Wolfson, S., & McLeer, S. V. (1990). Diagnosis of panic disorder in prepubertal children. *Journal of the American Academy of Child and Adolescent Psychiatry*, *29*, 782–784.

Walkup, J. T., Labellarte, M. J., & Ginsburg, G. S. (2002). The pharmacological treatment of childhood anxiety disorders. *International Review of Psychiatry*, *14*, 135–142.

Warren, S. L., Huston, L., Egeland, B., & Sroufe, L. A. (1997). Child and adolescent anxiety disorders and early attachment. *Journal of the American Academy of Child and Adolescent Psychiatry*, *36*, 637–644.

Waters, E., Vaughn, B. E., Posada, G., & Kondo-Ikemura, K. (1995). Caregiving, cultural, and cognitive perspectives on secure-base behavior and working models: New growing points of attachment theory and research. *Mono-*

graphs of the Society for Research in Child Development, 60(2–3, Serial No. 244).

Waters, V. (1979). *Color us rational.* New York: Institute for Rational Living.

Waters, V. (1980). *Rational stories for children.* New York: Institute for Rational Emotive Therapy.

Weems, C. F., Silverman, W. K., & La Greca, A. M. (2000). What do youth referred for anxiety problems worry about? Worry and its relation to anxiety and anxiety disorders in children and adolescents. *Journal of Abnormal Child Psychology, 28,* 63–72.

Weller, E. B., Weller, R. A., Fristad, M. A., Rooney, M. T., & Schecter, J. (2000). Children's Interview for Psychiatric Syndromes (ChIPS). *Journal of the American Academy of Child and Adolescent Psychiatry, 39,* 76–84.

Wijeratne, C., & Manicavasagar, V. (2003). Separation anxiety in the elderly. *Journal of Anxiety Disorders, 17,* 695–702.

Wittchen, H. U., Reed, V., & Kessler, R. C. (1998). The relationship of agoraphobia and panic in a community sample of adolescents and young adults. *Archives of General Psychiatry, 55,* 1017–1024.

Wolpe, J. (1992). *The practice of behavior therapy.* New York: Pergamon Press.

Yeragani, V., Meiri, P., Balon, R., Patel, H., & Pohl, R. (1989). History of separation anxiety in patients with panic disorder and depression and normal controls. *Acta Psychiatrica Scandinavica, 79,* 550–556.

Young, J. E. (1990). *Cognitive therapy for personality disorders: A schema-focused approach.* Sarasota, FL: Professional Resource Exchange.

Zarb, J. M. (1992). *Cognitive-behavioral assessment and therapy with adolescents.* New York: Brunner/Mazel.

Zitrin, C. M., Klein, D. F., Woerner, M. G., & Ross, D. C. (1983). Treatment of phobias: I. Comparisons of imipramine hydrochloride and placebo. *Archives of General Psychiatry, 40,* 125–138.

Zitrin, C. M., & Ross, D. C. (1988). Early separation anxiety and adult agoraphobia. *Journal of Nervous and Mental Disease, 176,* 621–625.

Index